Who Has Seen a Blood Sugar?

Also Available from the American College of Physicians

American College of Physicians Home Care Guide for Cancer

Common Diagnostic Tests: Use and Interpretation, Second edition

Common Screening Tests

Computers in Clinical Practice: Managing Patients, Information, and Communication

Diagnostic Strategies for Common Medical Problems

Drug Prescribing in Renal Failure: Dosing Guidelines for Adults, Third edition

Ethical Choices: Case Studies for Medical Practice

Guide for Adult Immunization, Third edition

Medical Care of the Nursing Home Resident: What Physicians Need To Know

Who Has Seen a Blood Sugar?

Reflections on Medical Education

Frank Davidoff, MD,
Editor, *Annals of Internal Medicine*
American College of Physicians
Philadelphia, Pennsylvania

with

Susan Deutsch, MD
Kathleen L. Egan, PhD
Jack Ende, MD

American College of Physicians
Philadelphia, Pennsylvania

A|C|P

Acquisitions Editor: Mary K. Ruff
Director of Book and Journal Publishing: Pamela Fried
Administrator, Book Publishing: Diane M. McCabe
Production Supervisor: Patricia C. Walter
Production Editor: Vicki Hoenigke
Interior Design: Larry Didona
Cover Design: Larry Didona

Printed in the United States of America.
Composition by ACP Graphic Services.
Printing/binding by Capitol City Press.
Cover printed by Capitol City Press.

American College of Physicians
Independence Mall West
Sixth Street at Race
Philadelphia, PA 19106-1572

Library of Congress Cataloging in Publication Data

Davidoff, Frank, 1934-
   Who has seen a blood sugar? : reflections on medical education / Frank Davidoff, with Susan Deutsch, Kathleen Egan, Jack Ende.
     232 p.   cm.
   Collection of articles originally published in ACP Observer, Mar. 1992–Nov. 1995.
   Includes index.
   ISBN: 0-943126-47-9
   1. Medical education—Miscellanea. I. Deutsch, Susan. II. Egan, Kathleen. III. Ende, Jack. IV. Title.
   [DNLM: 1. Education, Medical—collected works. 2. Teaching—collected works. 3. Learning—collected works. W 18 D2605w 1996]
   R740.D38 1996
   610'.71—dc20
   DNLM/DLC
   for Library of Congress
                                                                        96-2019
                                                                        CIP

96 97 98 99 00 01 / 9 8 7 6 5 4 3 2 1

For Jon, *the past*

For Ann, *the present*

For Jenny and Nina, *the future*

Who has seen the wind?
    Neither you nor I;
But when the trees bow down their heads
    The wind is passing by.

CHRISTINA ROSSETTI
Who Has Seen the Wind?

CONTRIBUTORS

Susan Deutsch, MD
Senior Associate for Education and Career Development
Division of Education
American College of Physicians
Philadelphia, Pennsylvania

Kathleen L. Egan, PhD
Senior Associate for Research and Development
Division of Education
American College of Physicians
Philadelphia, Pennsylvania

Jack Ende, MD
Professor of Medicine
Associate Dean and Director
for Network and Primary Care Education
University of Pennsylvania
Philadelphia, Pennsylvania

These essays appeared in *ACP Observer* in the following issues, except as noted.

CONTENTS

PART *TWO*   FEELINGS

PART *THREE* SYMBIOSIS

PREFACE

The pieces in this book were written during my years as Senior Vice President for Education at the American College of Physicians. Most of them appeared originally in the College's monthly newspaper, *ACP Observer*, between March 1992 and November 1995. These years were also the time when we all were trying to launch ourselves into the new information age. As a result, my electronic mail address appeared with each column, and readers were asked to send me comments and feedback electronically. Some columns produced no reaction at all; others led to extensive and helpful comment, criticism, and debate, sometimes lasting for weeks. The group that responded, via both electronic mail and an ACP electronic forum, wasn't large, but people weren't shy. Along the way came several suggestions that I collect the columns in a single place. This book of essays, revised and slightly expanded from the pieces in the *Observer*, is the result.

FOREWORD

*I*magine, if you will, that you have wandered into the book-lined study of a friend who seems to have interests very similar to yours; imagine, too, that he seems to have much more time than you do to read broadly about topics only distantly related to those you share. Further imagine that he has a gift for pithy, lucid summaries of such material that make you feel you understand it even if you won't have time to read it yourself; now imagine that he brings remarkable insights from these outside readings and that, as a result, almost everything you read about seems different than it did before—and that you thus learn something new on almost every page about things you have been living with and thinking about for years.

Assume now that in another part of the same study you see a remarkable conjunction of things too often separated. The cognitive side of your shared universe is illuminated by a combination of informal eloquence and accessible quantification. But in the next breath the author reminds you that medicine is never purely cognitive but always involves a feeling being who owns the illness and whose judgments about it and disability from it are unique, inviolable, and as important as any other clinical feature.

Surrounded by such delicacies, one is tempted to indulge continuously because it's as hard to stop as it is to eat one peanut. But here I have some advice for anyone lucky enough to fall into such another's study. Restrict yourself to no more than two or three of the items at a time. Then close the book, sit back, and think about what you've just read. Don't let its apparent simplicity fool you. Ponder each item and realize how dramatically, if effortlessly, your familiar world is being turned upside down. Realize that you have just been changed and that you're going to greet your next patient differently; that you will redo lectures you've given for years; that you will start your next ward rounds in a way that will surprise and delight your residents. Relish that you're positioned to think about learning rather than teaching.

If you've done all this without being observed, back out of the study and be thrilled that the person you've been spying on is at the very center of American medical thinking. Editor of the principal journal of internal medicine, *Annals of Internal Medicine,* and regular contributor to *ACP Observer,* Frank Davidoff has the gift of speaking publicly but somehow directly to you as an individual.

And then realize that you don't have to imagine or hope for any of these delicious treats. They exist, and here they are in one gem of a book.

DANIEL D. FEDERMAN, MD
HARVARD MEDICAL SCHOOL

ACKNOWLEDGMENTS

*U*ntil I came to write these acknowledgments, I had no idea how many people helped me put all of this together. Now I do, and the acknowledgments that appear in books make much more sense to me than they did before. I owe special thanks to the following people.

First, to John Ball for his support at every turn and particularly for his steadfast belief in the value of sabbaticals. Irwin Schatz, John Benson, and Jock Murray gave important additional encouragement along the way.

Then, to the editors of *ACP Observer*, Bob Spanier and Paula Katz, who got me started on these pieces, kept me going, and were enthusiastic at every step. I greatly appreciate the editorial work of Jan Corwin Enger of the *Observer* staff, and Susan Perry's help in assembling the book was indispensable.

And to my collaborators on several essays, who deserve much of the credit for those efforts. Working with Jack Ende, I learned to think about curriculum in entirely new ways, from the ground up, as it were; seeing a new mental model of curriculum take shape was a heady experience. Kathy Egan's hard, creative work on the Commitment for Change technique is undoubtedly the best to date. Susan Deutsch has been a leader in community-based teaching, and it shows.

A great many other people helped in a great many other ways; I've tried to remember them all but am sure I haven't. The ones I do remember include (more or less in alphabetical order):

Etta Berner, for her input on basic science; Caroline Blonde, for her insights into the mind of the murder mystery fan; Linda Bouchard and Mary Houts for sharing their knowledge of the Suzuki method; Iain Chalmers and Lelia Duley, for their patience and help in understanding the essential nature of the Cochrane Collaboration; Clifton Cleaveland, for inviting me to the Tennessee Reading Retreat, and for his many insightful, passionate disquisitions; Steve Clyman, for many good discussions about computer-based examinations; Leonore Davidoff, for pointing me to good material on manners; Dan Duffy, Wendy Levinson, Mack Lipkin, Penny Williamson, and other colleagues and friends too numerous to mention at the American Academy on Physician and Patient, for their unflagging energy in promoting the understanding and teaching of medical interviewing, and for including me in their efforts; Deborah Jones, for sharing her experience with and her writing on the Commitment for Change strategy; Harry Kimball and Paul Ramsey, for sharing their knowledge of the recertification process; Christine Laine and Tom Delbanco, for their important collaborations on patient-centered care; John Noble, for his enduring interest in the teaching legacy of David Seegal, and for his assistance in tracking down references on it; John Parboosingh, for his generous explanations of the Maintenance of Competence Program; Bob Rippey, who opened up for me the universe of confidence testing; Bob Spena, Jerry Osheroff, and Larry Blonde, for an incredible number of interesting, important discussions about medical informatics, medical computing, and clinical information management; Paula Stillman, for sharing her enormous experience with standardized patients; Geoffrey Williams, for introducing me to self-determination theory and convincing me that it makes sense; and Tony Voytovich, a friend and colleague, for teaching me much.

Finally, some general thanks: to the staff in the Education Division of the American College of Physicians for putting up with me while I produced these essays every month, and to several of the Education Division staff members, particularly Theresa Kanya and Kathy Egan for reading them critically; to the many readers of the *Observer* who took the time and trouble to comment; to the Rockefeller Foundation for the opportunity to revise and expand the work at the Villa Serbelloni in Bellagio; and to Ann, for unfailingly being my best critic.

The people mentioned above, and others not mentioned, are responsible for much that is good and useful in these pieces; I am, of course, entirely responsible for any shortcomings.

INTRODUCTION

A few words on what these essays aren't. First, they aren't about pedagogy. Pedagogy—in the sense of educational method and technique—is obviously important, but there is already an existing literature on pedagogy (and its more "grownup" counterpart, andragogy), some of it quite good (and some of it mind-numbingly dull). Besides, despite a career covering nearly forty years as a medical education watcher and teacher, I acquired no special expertise in pedagogy, so I had little to contribute to the topic.

Second, they aren't a treatise. The idea of the *Updates* was not to focus on a single theme, but to explore whatever there was about medical education that seemed interesting, exciting, frustrating, misguided, or generally worthy of thought and comment. This, of course, was cheating, because there is an educational aspect to almost everything and anything. There was, consequently, no real limit on what I could explore and, consequently, the essays are eclectic, touching on a wide variety of things—disease severity, efficiency, aphorisms, quitting smoking, murder mysteries—not traditionally considered "educational." And there seemed to be no end to the sources— music, poetry, mathematics, fiction—of potential insight about medicine and medical education. I make no apologies for this; on the contrary, these are exactly the kinds of things that, to me, make medical education endlessly interesting, as it should be.

Third, they aren't scholarly. Every essay does provide selected, key references that tie it to useful published work; every one tries to be internally coherent; and they all are grounded in data, whenever possible. But on the whole, the essays don't build systematically on other bodies of thought. Rather, I tried to "write what I know," about ideas from my own medical and educational experience that "jelled" things for me, about concepts and thinking that helped me make sense of things.

What they are is explorations, reflections, essays. There is no shortage of superb modern models, from medicine, science, and elsewhere, for the writing of essays. While I didn't consciously draw on any particular model, I know that I owe a debt to many, including Lewis Thomas, for his ability to fuse lucid thought with limpid language; Stephen Jay Gould, for his ability to take insights from the most unlikely sources; and Susan Sontag, for the sheer power of her intellect. M.F.K. Fisher's gift of writing broadly about the important things in life while seeming to write about the microcosm of food was an important influence.

Medicine is, of course, an extraordinarily mysterious and demanding profession—a complex mixture of biology, technology, social and behavioral science, ethics, and humanism. Even at its scientific best, medicine is *always* a social act. There is therefore no shortage of things to explore and to reflect on in an education system that takes smart, idealistic students, initiates them into these mysteries, and transforms them into the medical professionals who would be almost unrecognizable to their premedical selves. Writing these essays was an opportunity to cut through some of the myths and the conventions, the distancing and the isolation, the jargon and the rhetoric that surround the medical education system, and get to the heart—or the gut realities, if you prefer—of the matter. It was an opportunity to examine unexamined assumptions. To move past hard questions such as "How can we teach basic science better?" to harder questions such as "Is basic science necessary?" To explore some of the more intriguing and subtle aspects of medicine, such as uncertainty, confidence, interest, and the nature of explanations. To weave together the thinking of others and my own perceptions, creating new patterns, finding linkages, bridging gaps.

They also exhort. Things worth commenting on, in medical education as elsewhere, are sometimes especially admirable but more often especially problematic. It is, however, only a short step from commenting to sermonizing, all too easy to become an armchair admiral. In my view, the U.S. medical education system in the 1990s needs and deserves serious thought and work, but it is an extraordinary system, well worth preserving; it is not one that needs to be torn down and built up again from scratch. While there was no way to keep these essays from being prescriptive, I did try therefore to avoid hand-wringing and did try wherever possible to lay out concrete ideas on how things might be seen differently, suggestions for how they might be made better.

In going back over four years worth of effort, I also came to realize that, despite the lack of a conscious unifying theme, the essays are linked into a kind of network. Or, more to the point, they cluster loosely into four groups, starting with the most narrowly focused and inward domain of intellectual work, working outward through the emotional, affective territory that surrounds it, then broadening further to the "symbiosis" between these two domains and, finally, out into the social, political, and economic context in which these all reside, and I've grouped the essays accordingly.

The first group, then, deals primarily with several kinds of mental models. Some we now work with in medicine and medical education; others, such as the concepts of predictive value, confidence testing, scoreable problem lists, and experiential curriculum, seem to me to be fundamental improvements over models that are now commonly used.

The second group gets into the topic of feelings, something that is rarely given serious, conscious attention in connection with medical education. When feeling and emotion are acknowledged at all, they are seen pretty much as an annoyance and a distraction, in much the same way that turbulence and other nonlinear systems behavior were viewed as annoyances in the physical sciences over the years. However, once it was recognized that those previously baffling anomalies have a higher-order regularity, a meaning of their own, they became the object of intense, creative study that ultimately led to the development of the theory of chaos and a major transformation of the way people look at the physical world. Interest, belief, confidence, satisfaction, educational value, manners, and uncertainty are the nonlinear, turbulent behaviors of medical education. They deserve, in my view, the kind of creative thought that has been devoted to nonlinear systems in physics, and the same careful attention that the intellectual side of medicine now receives. Improvement in our ability to deal with the affective side of things medical and educational carries enormous potential payoff for both medicine and education.

But each of these broad domains—thinking and feeling—by itself is not "the problem," either in medical education or medicine. In fact, it seems to me that "the problem" (if there is a single, over-arching problem) is the tendency for one domain to overshadow the other, or, stated the other way around, our inability to bring the two together in a "symbiosis." In this I have been influenced by the social geographer Jane Jacobs who, in a powerful Socratic essay called *Systems of Survival* (1), argues that human affairs are governed on a macro level by two "moral syndromes," the commercial and the guardian. According to Jacobs, the two syndromes have evolved from different origins and along different historical courses. Each is constituted of a set of a dozen or more deeply held values that is not only different from but also contrary to the other. For example, the commercial (i.e., business, entrepreneurial) syndrome places great value on qualities such as efficiency, innovation, competition, thrift, and openness; whereas the guardian (i.e., military, church, state) syndrome places similarly great value on tradition, prowess, ceremony, ostentation, obedience, honor, and largesse.

Jacobs argues further that both syndromes in some form are essential for a sane and civilized society, indeed that social systems in which one syndrome dominates, in which one takes over the functions best dealt with by the other, become what she calls "monstrous hybrids." Examples of monstrous hybrids include the virtually total dominance by the guardian syndrome under the Soviet regime (government bureaucracy taking over the entire commercial enterprise), and the virtually total dominance by the commercial syndrome in Nazi Germany (the efficiency of the commercial sector applied to governmental and social policy).

According to Jacobs's view, then, the bringing together of the two syndromes in a balanced and carefully controlled way—a "symbiosis" in her terms—is essential if the entire social system is not to become a disaster. Jacobs doesn't pretend that such a synthesis or symbiosis is easy; true symbiosis involves a kind of controlled tension between the two syndromes that is difficult to achieve in the first place and even harder to maintain over the long run. But she does argue that it is possible— and that it is essential.

While medicine doesn't replicate exactly in microcosm the broad sweep of human affairs, it does seem to me that medicine contains within itself two analogous moral syndromes of its own, the cognitive (intellectual, scientific) and the affective (emotional, humanistic), each with its own set of strong values and powerful assumptions. Medicine and, consequently, medical education arguably have also created a few monstrous hybrids of their own, including the following: the pronounced (and much maligned) skew toward subspecialty medicine at the expense of generalized medicine; the powerful but ambiguous role of basic science in medicine, and the related preoccupation with high-tech medicine, particularly in the apparent absence of either the will or the tools to manage this aspect of the profession as well as it should be managed; the dominance of authoritarianism over authoritativeness in many parts of medicine; the disdain for medical teaching as both a discipline and a career; and the isolation of the theory and practice of medical teaching from the rest of the educational world, and from the wider humanistic and cultural world beyond that. At the margin, medicine finds itself increasingly hung up on the fundamental moral question of whether it is mainly a business, and hence part of the commercial syndrome, or a profession, and hence part of the guardian syndrome; and undergraduate medical education faces the parallel dilemma of whether it is mainly a trade school or a graduate school. Both reflect the very dilemma Jacobs identifies as intrinsic to the larger social world.

The third group of essays thus includes topics that can be seen as elements in a symbiosis: concrete, direct links between the cognitive and the affective; between thinking and feeling; between science and humanism. The development of rigorous techniques for assessing clinical skills; the differences between education and training; severity as a link between "disease" and "illness," the science of understanding and teaching about uncertainty, the difference between knowledge and confidence, and related topics all seemed to me to belong to this group.

Finally, the broader social and political and economic context in which medical education happens is represented in the fourth group, largely by the issues surrounding continuing medical education (CME). For while the broader context obviously affects medical school and residency training, those two segments of medical education exist in a world that is, relatively speaking, protected from the cross-currents of the larger one. CME, in contrast, is right out there in the marketplace, as attested to by its "pre-Flexnerian" character, if by nothing else; that is, CME is only distantly linked to the academic community; it varies widely (if not wildly) in nature and quality; and it is highly proprietary, principally with regard to its intimate and powerful links to medical industry.

Is there, even implicitly, a deeper underlying theme to these essays? Readers will have to judge for themselves. But to the extent that there is one, it may be reflected in the book's title, *Who Has Seen a Blood Sugar?* The essay by that title evoked more interest and comment than any other and has apparently, therefore, touched on something fundamental. This something seems to be the recognition that both the power and the frailty of medicine are rooted in its ability to shape the invisible world. Sick patients themselves are highly visible and tangible, but medicine has always managed to skip rapidly beyond these realities and into the realms of invisible forces, once the spiritual and the demonic, now the biomedical and the mechanistic.

Medicine was once part of religion, and healing was once (and still is, in most parts of the world) clearly and explicitly part of spiritual experience. To the enormous benefit of patients, science moved medicine away from its doctrinaire relationship with religion. But in the process, medicine has come to believe that it has left the invisible world behind; that it now deals only with the *hard* realities—the data, the observations, the images, and the like. But medicine hasn't left the invisible world behind at all; it has only moved into a new and different invisible world of its own, which has taken on an enormously compelling reality, and in which medicine now literally lives. Since this is, however, a reality we have shaped, we can, to the extent it doesn't work, reshape it. If these essays help shape medical reality so it is even a little more graceful, a little more effective than it has been, that will be more than is given to most.

REFERENCE

1. **Jacobs J.** Systems of Survival. A Dialogue on the Moral Foundations of Commerce and Politics. New York: Vintage Books/Random House, 1992.

PART ONE

MENTAL MODELS

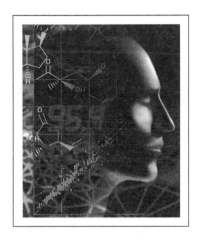

CHAPTER 1

Teaching Files and Textbook Examples

~

The Case of the Classic Case

*T*he patient was a middle-aged man. Slightly bewildered by the presence of so many medical students—the twenty or so of us who had been summoned to his bedside from our many scattered teaching services—he listened quietly as our instructor pointed out the puffy, coarse features, the croaking voice, the slowed movements, the "hung" reflexes—virtually every clinical finding of a classic case of myxedema. In nearly forty years of medicine since that day, a quarter of it in endocrinology, I've never forgotten him. And while I've seen many other patients with myxedema since then, I've never seen another patient so florid, so classic.

The demonstration of classic or textbook examples (paradigms, prototypical cases) is a hallowed tradition in clinical teaching, at least in teaching medical diagnosis. Classic cases are commonly collected into teaching files, a resource particularly beloved by people who work with medical images—radiologists, pathologists, endoscopists, and the like—because, understandably, picture-perfect images have so much intrinsic appeal. But, of course, classic cases also turn up in verbal form in grand rounds and teaching conferences and clinicopathologic conferences; in textbooks (hence the expression "textbook case"); and in many other education-related venues, including medical examination questions.

For all that they are memorable, classic cases are also rare; both certainly proved true for the case of classic myxedema encountered during my student days. This important paradox is underscored by the traditional publications on diagnosis—those papers, more common in previous eras, that describe in meticulous detail the diagnostic findings of a particular disease in a group or series of patients. The tables in these papers almost always tell us that, while a few findings were present in 100 percent of the group, many others were present in a middling proportion, say, 25 percent to 75 percent, of patients, and still others were unusual, each occurring in just a few patients in the group.

Now, it takes some doing to think about data like these in reverse, that is, to translate information about groups back into the findings as they occur in individual patients. When you make that translation, however, it becomes obvious that it is the rare patient, statistically speaking, who can be expected to demonstrate every finding in the book. This rare patient is the "classic case," the patient whose findings most fully typify the disease (which, not coincidentally, is likely to be the patient with the most long-standing, hence perhaps also the most neglected or untreated, disease).

We have here, then, the makings of a pedagogical conundrum: the tradition of *using case examples you may never see again to teach about diseases you are likely to see every day.* For, on the one hand, what could be more natural, more logical than to teach from classic examples? Or, stated the other way around, who would want to teach from the atypical case, the bizarre example, the exception? From the learner's point of view, the classic case is, after all, likely to be the most memorable case, and the creation of memorable mental structures, models, or scripts is a crucial part of learning. On the other hand, as we've seen above, the "classic case" approach to clinical teaching is itself unrepresentative, even bizarre. For some mysterious reason, using extreme examples makes us uncomfortable. Perhaps the source of this discomfort is because at bottom it's reminiscent of the "best-in-show" mentality associated with dogs or cattle, where a champion is the exemplar of all the features that define the breed—and as clinicians and teachers, we don't like to think we operate in that kind of competitive, outlier mode.

As a way of teaching diagnostic medicine, the use of full-blown, classic cases raises a number of interesting and important questions. Since their power lies principally in being memorable, the use of classic cases may be an efficient way of imprinting beginners with sets of diagnostic information. For clinicians with significant experience, however, the recognition of classic cases is generally a "no-brainer." Encountering a classic case may be a pleasure for an expert clinician, but the real challenge for expert clinicians lies rather in recognizing the subtle, less-than-classic patient and in the Sherlock Holmes–like unraveling of the baffling case. More to the point, both everyday practice and the published diagnostic literature described above teach us that most patients with a given disease in fact present in less-than-classic, nonspecific ways, most with only a few findings or even a single one. There is often an even bigger reservoir of asymptomatic patients with the earliest stages of the disease, detectable only by some more sensitive means of testing, which is of course what screening is all about.

Thus, we have now framed the reverse pedagogical conundrum: *The patients you are numerically most likely to see every day are not likely to be classic cases of the disease;* or, stated more concisely, the typical patient is atypical. As you probe beneath the surface of this conundrum, two further lessons emerge. First, it is the day-to-day experience of caring for ordinary patients, not the rare, once-in-a-lifetime classic patient encounter, that provides the most important opportunity for diagnostic learning at an advanced level—that is, recognizing the subtle, the nonspecific, the nonclassic findings of disease.

And second, time is a critical dimension in case-based diagnostic teaching. For the simple reality is that many cases are not initially recognized as classic, but rather identified as such only after a good deal of diagnostic evidence is assembled. The diagnostic process almost invariably unfolds over time, with many twists and turns, tantalizing leads, and frustrating dead ends along its path. Yet in formal teaching exercises, the case history is traditionally presented entirely, giving learners a kind of bird's eye, after-the-fact version of the diagnostic process. Compiled case histories like these, in which the events are crunched together into a single seamless scenario, may be more classic, but they lack the clinical fidelity of events as they actually play out over time. Presented after the fact, such cases oversimplify and distort the reality of learning and practicing clinical diagnosis.

It is precisely the ability to reconstruct the time dimension (at least partly) that adds teaching value to the particular species of clinical problem-solving exercises championed by Jerome Kassirer and his colleagues (1,2). They accomplish this reconstruction through the simple stratagem of presenting chunks of information for discussion in sequence, as they emerged over time, rather than in the traditional cumulative snapshot.

But there's more. Consider now the diagnostic dilemma of a 24-year-old woman who presents with the relatively rapid onset of a red and exquisitely tender big toe. Reasoning from cases like this, Custers and colleagues (3) in the Netherlands have argued that diagnostic information falls into several general categories, most importantly 1) enabling conditions (or "context" information, including age, gender, environmental and family history, and the like); and 2) clinical consequences (which include signs and symptoms, and clinical and laboratory findings).

In the above patient, the presenting clinical consequence, podagra, is entirely typical (classic) for gout, but the enabling conditions (age, gender) are atypical (nonclassic). Conversely, in the case of a 55-year-old man with hypertension who drinks a good deal of alcohol and presents with bilateral red and tender wrists, the enabling conditions are classic for gout, but the clinical consequences are not. Interestingly, the Dutch investigators have shown that experienced clinicians and medical students both rely on enabling conditions (information that is important in determining prior probabilities) in arriving at diagnoses, but experienced clinicians place significantly more weight on the typicality of enabling conditions than students do (3). (See Chapter 25, A Touch of Cancer.)

Thus, as much as we might wish otherwise, diagnostic information is not homogenous: a single case can be *partly* classic, *partly* not. Like it or not, learning advanced diagnostic skills involves learning not only how to manage subtle, nonspecific, nonclassic findings, but also how to combine and weigh dissonant information—that is, the typical and the atypical existing together within a single patient. Classic cases occupy an important niche in the medical education environment, but the niche turns out to be a small one, after all. What a pity. Classic cases are so clear, so recognizable, so memorable, so . . . classic. You'd think that on their merits they'd count for more in clinical teaching than they do, more than the ordinary or the subtle. But, by the same token, where would the challenge be if everything were a classic?

REFERENCES

1. **Kassirer JP, Kopelman RI.** Learning Clinical Reasoning. Baltimore, MD: Williams and Wilkins; 1991.
2. **Kassirer JP.** Clinical problem-solving: a new feature in the Journal. N Engl J Med. 1992;326:60-1.
3. **Custers EJM, Boshuizen HA, Schmidt HG.** The influence of typicality of case descriptions on subjective disease probability estimates. Presented at the Annual Meeting of the American Educational Research Association; April 12–16, 1993; Atlanta, GA.

CHAPTER 2

Information and Education

Filling in the Blanks

*T*he lab calls you with the latest results on your patient, Ms. Garfield, a woman in her 60s with class IV congestive failure, who is receiving treatment with digoxin, furosemide, and an angiotensin-converting enzyme (ACE) inhibitor. Her potassium level is 6.2.

What's just happened here? You might casually describe this transaction by saying you've *learned* that Ms. Garfield's potassium level is elevated. But have you really been educated, in some meaningful sense of the word, or were you given a piece of *information*? Suppose, now, that you sit down to read the latest issue of your favorite medical journal or that you attend grand rounds. Are these sources of education or of information? Are there really differences between the two? If so, what? Many signs indicate that there *are* differences: the very fact that the language contains two separate and specific terms for the two concepts; the assertion by Stephen Lock, the former editor of the *British Medical Journal*, that medical journals should both "inform and instruct" (1); and even the stated mission of the American College of Physicians of being "the principal education and information resource for internists."

A pragmatic view of this fundamental but complex problem is to think of information as *data that fill in the blanks in existing mental templates*. Looked at this way, a piece of information by itself carries little meaning; rather, it acquires meaning largely from the template into which it fits. Yet information thus narrowly defined carries no less weight for all that. The information content of the word "Yes," by itself, is trivial, but its impact is enormous when it fits into slots created by templates like: "Will you marry me?" or "Do I have cancer?"

Education, by contrast, is *the process that creates the templates.* Templates range from simple rule-based constructs, such as "If the serum potassium level is elevated, stop the ACE inhibitor, increase the diuretic, and recheck the potassium level," to more sophisticated structures, such as the pathophysiology of congestive failure and the clinical pharmacology of digitalis, diuretics, and ACE inhibitors, all the way to elaborate mental models at the cellular and molecular level.

The world presses in on us with enormous amounts of information. The principal challenge, therefore, is not how to get ahold of more information; on the contrary, the problem is how to filter information, fit it into the right slots, and keep it where it belongs. We have a pretty fair idea of how information "works." The more difficult question is "How does education work?" How, in effect, do the templates get constructed? One current view is that people acquire many of their working mental models—of the nature of things, of causality, of consequences—"naturally" and almost automatically, early in life and mostly through experiences outside formal schooling. Moreover, while these models are somewhat primitive or simplistic, they appear to work reasonably well for most people in dealing with most everyday problems and situations. For this reason, among others, these models are deeply rooted and, therefore, extremely resistant to change (2). (See Chapter 18, Who Has Seen A Blood Sugar?)

In this view, most formal education (perhaps better known as "schooling") appears intended to develop rote, ritualistic or conventional performances. To this end teachers dispense, and students acquire, thousands of chunks of information through memorization, teaching to the test, and the building of fragile pseudotemplates—mental constructs that serve their purpose well enough as long as learners are working in the right context: a classroom, a homework assignment, a test. Such information masquerading as education is, unfortunately, prone to rapid disuse atrophy. More importantly, pseudotemplates are of little help when learners are confronted with new situations—the kind of unfamiliar situations that require a deeper understanding, more flexibility, and the ability to apply knowledge quickly, appropriately, gracefully—what has been called "genuine," disciplinary, or expert level understanding (2). While there are, of course, exceptions, evidence strongly indicates that this bleak picture of formal education extends throughout the system, from the earliest years through college (and on into at least the first year or two of traditional medical school teaching); from the most resource-poor school systems to the best endowed ones; from the brightest to the most ordinary students; and from the distant past right up to the present day (3). (See Chapter 24, The Right Hand of Claude.)

Student resistance to acquiring elaborated, more sophisticated mental models certainly contributes to the picture. Importantly, however, it is now increasingly clear that students don't resist "genuine" learning because they are intimidated, confused, or just plain pig-headed. The evidence is this. First, the resistance appears to be partly biological in origin. The brain is called on to make refined discriminations with a sensory and processing apparatus that is, at bottom, grainy and coarse; it accomplishes this in many instances by using "hard-wired" search and processing mechanisms. The result is that "we are constantly deceived about the nature of the outside world because we interpret it in terms of the built-in . . . mechanism[s]" (4). The ability of these brain mechanisms to convert incomplete or ill-formed images and thoughts into completed but stereotypical, distorted, or biased ones is really quite dramatic (5,6).

Second, students misapply their deeply held but simplistic models in specific ways, depending on the nature of the subject (2,6). Thus, errors in science are most frequently due to the use of *misconceptions;* in mathematics, to rigid application of rules or *algorithms;* and in the arts and humanities, to *stereotyping* and *oversimplification* (2). Observations like these suggest that resistance to the changing of templates is due to a selective dissonance between each new mental model and a particular established belief rather than to a nonspecific, generalized "turning off."

While the demonstration of specific, recurring error patterns is in some ways discouraging, their recognition opens important alternative approaches to effective teaching and learning, in the spirit of self-improvement, or *kaizen* (Japanese), where "every defect is a treasure." Moreover, other recent investigations of the structure of knowledge—the character of descriptions (7) and of consciousness itself (8)—as abstruse as they seem at first, now provide important clues to ways in which mental models are built and changed; pictures, in effect, of how "genuine" education works. The central concept here is the nature of *explanations,* that is, accounting for the behavior of one thing in terms of others. Explanations in science are usually, but not always, "reductionistic"; they link more complex things to others that are regarded as less complex or that occupy lower levels in a hierarchy of "complete descriptions," as, for example, the explanation of clinical findings in a disease such as phenylketonuria in terms of mutation in a single gene (7).

But while many important and complex properties of higher-level entities can be rigorously understood (explained), in the literal sense, by a combination of lower-level attributes (e.g., water, which can be "understood" as a combination of hydrogen and oxygen atoms), it is equally important to recognize that other higher-level properties (e.g., excited states of electrons; chronic fatigue; societal violence) cannot. Or, stated the other way around, a theory that is sufficient for complete description at one level of organization is not, and need not be, capable of predicting properties that emerge at the next, higher level—the concept of so-called "emergent properties." Emergent properties make the construction of mental models much more complicated, but also much more interesting (7).

Other important asymmetric explanatory relationships also emerge from the hierarchy of descriptions. Thus, while some higher-level entities (e.g., mice) can be partly understood (explained) by reference to the properties of molecules and atoms, it doesn't always work the other way around, that is, it isn't possible literally to "understand" molecules in terms of mice. In other hierarchies it is possible to understand a lower-level entity (e.g., clockwork) only in terms of a higher-level entity (i.e., human beings, with their concepts of time and of mechanical engineering), while the converse is not true: The higher-level entity (human beings) can't be understood in terms of the lower-level entity (clockwork), except in a metaphorical sense.

For all its explanatory power, it is doubtful whether the descriptive hierarchy of the real world, with its emergent properties, its asymmetrical linkages, and the vast amount of information it still lacks, by itself can ever be the sole basis for creating adequate mental models, that is, deep understanding; it is simply too complex, too abstract. It is here that a different species of explanatory linkage—namely, metaphor—becomes an important and, at times, essential tool in understanding, particularly at the highest levels of the descriptive hierarchy. In fact, the psychologist Julian Jaynes goes so far as to state that (8)

> Understanding a thing is to arrive at a metaphor for that thing by substituting something more familiar to us. And the feeling of familiarity is the feeling of understanding.

It is certainly true, in medicine and elsewhere, that the meaning of a complex phenomenon often remains opaque until someone says "Think of it this way. It's like . . ." At an important level, illness itself can probably only be understood through metaphor (9). And, at the extreme, understanding in poetry works largely through metaphor:

"The moon was a ghostly galleon, tossed upon cloudy seas. . . ."

However we define information and education, the practice of medicine clearly requires them both. According to our pragmatic definitions, most medical discourse as we know it today, including medical education and medical journalism, is made up of a blend of information and education, sometimes more of one, sometimes more of the other. This seems inevitable and not necessarily a bad thing. At the same time, an expanded understanding of the difference between the two, of how mental models are built, and, hence, how explanations work, makes clear just how much more there is to "genuine" education than simply filling in the blanks.

REFERENCES

1. **Lock S.** A Difficult Balance: Editorial Peer Review in Medicine. Philadelphia: ISI Press; 1986.
2. **Gardner H.** The Unschooled Mind: How Children Think and How Schools Should Teach. New York: Basic Books; 1991.
3. **Koman K.** Newton, one-on-one: a new way of teaching physics. Harvard Magazine. 1995;97:18-9.
4. **Bronowski J.** The Origins of Knowledge and Imagination. New Haven, CT: Yale University Press; 1978.
5. **Edwards B.** Drawing on the Right Side of the Brain. New York: St Martin; 1988.
6. **Kahneman D, Slovic P, Tversky A,** eds. Judgment Under Uncertainty: Heuristics and Biases. New York: Cambridge University Press; 1982.
7. **Blois MS.** Information and Medicine: The Nature of Medical Descriptions. Berkeley, CA: University of California Press; 1984:56.
8. **Jaynes J.** The Origin of Consciousness in the Breakdown of the Bicameral Mind. Boston: Houghton Mifflin Co.; 1990.
9. **Sontag S.** Illness as Metaphor. New York: Farrar, Straus and Giroux; 1978.

CHAPTER 3

Music Lessons

The Learning of Medical Informatics

*I*nterest in medical informatics is growing exponentially, both in the United States and abroad. But despite all the interest and enthusiasm, the general experience is that learning medical informatics remains a serious challenge (1).

One problem right up front is that even the term *informatics* itself is obscure, meaning a variety of different things to different people (2). Most people who hear the word *informatics* immediately think "computers," which is understandable, perhaps, given the current obsession with that technology. But that view has the definition of the term backwards: A computer is as dumb as a radiator, a powerful tool, to be sure, but *only* a tool for managing information. Terms such as *information science* and *clinical information management* come much closer to expressing what the subject is all about (3). Moreover, as the novelty of computers—color graphics, the magic of "click-and-drag," the dazzle of the Windows environment, the universe of the information superhighway—begins to fade, even the most dedicated medical computer users recognize at some level that medical computing is less suited for dealing with the exotic and the cutting edge than it is for managing the messy and mundane, the everyday tasks of medical practice.

What is new and exciting, however, about the dawning medical informatics revolution is the emergence of the powerful, if somewhat abstract, notion that *information* is really what lies at the heart of medicine. (See Chapter 23, The Technologies of Education.) The revolution probably began quietly in the late 1960s with Lawrence Weed, MD, who taught us that the way we represent information about our patients in the written medical record is not just an epiphenomenon of care but, in fact, defines the reality of those patients' illnesses and of the entire care process.

The Weed System, or Problem-Oriented Medical Record, is often equated with one of its component parts, the SOAP format (Subjective, Objective, Assessment, and Plan). But the most truly revolutionary feature of the Problem-Oriented Medical Record is not the SOAP format at all, but the Master Problem List—a numbered and titled list of the medical issues confronting patients and their physicians (4). (See Chapter 5, The Voytovich Solution.) Indeed, legend has it that Weed did not consider the SOAP format as a central feature of the Problem-Oriented Medical Record at all and never intended it to be used in ordinary, written or typed medical records. Rather, he originally conceived of it as a specific technique for classifying the free text of progress notes so they could be entered into a computerized version of the medical record. It isn't surprising, therefore, that the SOAP format has proven cumbersome to use in written records. And unfortunately, this misapplication of a secondary element of Weed's powerful concept has probably inhibited more than it has encouraged widespread use of the Problem-Oriented Medical Record.

But the fat was in the fire. Weed had opened our eyes not only to the richness of information but, more importantly, to the terrible disorder in those old "source-oriented" records. Important information got lost in them, priorities were unclear, key data were hard to track, and communication was difficult. Worst of all, source-orientation made it nearly impossible to realize the full dynamic potential of medical records.

Early Problem-Oriented Medical Record enthusiasts were convinced that the new system would somehow itself improve the practice of medicine. The realists suspected that using the Problem-Oriented Medical Record, for all its power, was not like waving a magic wand but rather like turning on a light in a messy room: It simply makes cleaning up much easier. In effect, Weed showed us that good medical information management, like good housekeeping, defines a place for all information and puts all information in its place, and that good information management is the sine qua non of good medicine.

Most of all, Weed convinced us that the record information system needs, in Vince Lombardi's immortal words to the Green Bay Packers, to "do the simple things well." Computers can certainly help in creating and using a well-structured medical record system, since computers are extremely good at certain simple tasks people generally have trouble with—for example, storing, sorting, retrieving, and displaying information. But the core of a truly effective record system is not the computer on which it might reside, but a rational design that flows from the information needs of patients, physicians, nurses, and the others who matter in the care system; exemplary medical records certainly exist on paper. And despite the ballyhoo about the potential and power of "the computerized medical record," few such systems are in use as of the mid-1990s. Can it be that the design of most computer-based medical records systems developed to date reflects the interests and needs of computer scientists, accountants, and administrators more than those of physicians and their patients?

Over time, the basic rightness of Weed's message has been underscored in many interesting ways, the most graphic being the advent of electronic medical literature searching. In principle, searching the medical literature isn't all that difficult. Any one of us can flip through a few bound volumes of medical journals in the local medical library and even work our way through a few years of the paper version of *Index Medicus,* to come up with answers to at least some of our clinical questions—and many of us were brought up in medicine doing just that. Even the basic principle of electronic literature searching is simple; all it does is what doctors do all the time: look things up in journals and books.

So why all the fuss about electronic literature searching? Because the electronic system does this simple thing so extraordinarily *well.* Six or seven million references searched in a few seconds, instead of a few dozen references searched in a few hours. The jet plane versus the horse. No contest.

Electronic literature searching is the most mature and powerful of the new medical information systems. But it is not a perfect system: It is not all that easy to learn, often yielding no references at all or, contrariwise, an overabundance of them, and producing at best citations "in the raw"—that is, without quality filters of any kind. It cannot be entirely a coincidence that hard evidence for the clinical effectiveness of electronic searching has been slow to accumulate (5–7). And conversely, it should come as no surprise that the real advances in the accuracy and effectiveness of electronic literature searching appear to originate not in technological improvements but in better understanding of the structure of information, hence better design of the search process (8). (See Chapter 23, The Technologies of Education.)

In the meantime, other improved medical information systems have appeared. For example, electronic networks, palmtop computers, and fax machines have created whole new universes of accessible, transmissible, and portable medical information. But the most successful of these systems are, again, those that make for "good housekeeping," largely because computers are best at the homely things that matter, like writing orders (9) and generating and posting reminders (10).

When it comes to "expert" information systems—computer-based clinical reasoning, decision analysis, pattern recognition, diagnostic support—the going for informatics has been tougher (11). Human minds still have the edge here, although expert systems are finding a place in clinical work, particularly now that people understand that these systems are best used as an extension and amplifier of the human mind, like a stethoscope or an x-ray, rather than as a medical oracle, which was the earlier expectation (12). And with this understanding comes the recognition that the extension and amplification of human minds lie more in the enormous ability of computers to structure, organize, sort, and compare information than in their ability to "reason" about it.

But if the essence of medical informatics lies in doing the simple things well; if much of what appears mystifying and terrifying about medical informatics turns out, like the Wizard of Oz, to be just an ordinary man behind the curtain, why is medical informatics so hard to teach and learn? One reason may be that complicated electronic equipment of any kind is intimidating. And despite the advent of the "mouse," much of the interaction with computers still requires the use of a keyboard, which is definitely a problem for nontypists.

But perhaps most difficult of all is the problem of trying to absorb the arcane and alien mysteries of the instrument—the hardware and software—*at the same time* you are trying to understand the structure of medical information itself: crucial but abstract matters like the limitations of medical terminology, the uses of a medical thesaurus, the reasons why literature searches are either insensitive or nonspecific, and the ongoing quirks and convolutions of medical records. To make things worse, most people learn about about computers, information, and informatics on their own, which makes it an isolating and lonely experience.

Perhaps musicians have something to teach us here. For most people, learning to play a musical instrument is a daunting challenge, comparable to learning medical informatics in at least two ways. First, playing a musical instrument, particularly a stringed instrument such as violin or cello, requires learning about a delicate, subtle instrument (the hardware), the complexities of notes and harmonies and rhythms (the software), and, ultimately, the inner mysteries of music and musicality. And second, people learn to play instruments, particularly strings, in isolation.

In 1933, Shinichi Suzuki came to grips with the problem of getting learners, particularly children, started on stringed instruments. He reasoned that much of the difficulty in this undertaking may be associated with learning both to handle the instrument *and* to read music at the same time, even suspecting that the two learning processes may actually interfere with one another. He reasoned further that since children learn to speak without knowing how to read, students should be able to learn to play instruments "by ear," without needing to read music. In fact, he reasoned, students should learn to play their instruments more quickly and easily if they are *not* required to learn to read music at the same time. According to the Suzuki method, therefore, students play a stringed instrument for some six years before they are allowed to read music; and they learn the music by listening to recordings and by singing. What's more, the Suzuki method requires a young learner's parents to attend the lessons, and pupils are regularly required to play for each other, first in small groups, then larger ones. Learning a stringed instrument thus becomes an intrinsically social, rather than an isolating, experience.

Computers are not violins, and even the best word-processing program is not Twinkle, Twinkle Little Star, much less Beethoven's Fifth, but there may be important lessons here for students of medical informatics nonetheless. Perhaps the learning of hardware (plus operating) systems should be disengaged from the learning of applications (software) in ways that help more people get started in medical computing. Perhaps learning medical informatics can be organized so that it is a live, connected, group activity, a social as much as an intellectual process. Perhaps the full potential of medical information systems can finally be realized, becoming the harmony and counterpoint, the full orchestral score, of medical care.

REFERENCES

1. **Williams JG, de Dombal FT, Knill-Jones R, Severs MP.** Royal College of Physicians Committee on Medical Information Technology. Collecting, communicating and using information: the educational issues: A report from the Royal College of Physicians Committee on Medical Information Technology. J R Coll Phys Lond. 1992;26:385-7.

2. **Shortliffe EH, Perreault LE, eds.** Medical Informatics: Computer Applications in Health Care. Reading, MA: Addison-Wesley; 1990.

3. **Blois MS.** Information and Medicine: The Nature of Medical Descriptions. Berkeley, CA: University of California Press; 1984.

4. **Weed LL.** Medical Records, Medical Education, and Patient Care. Chicago: Year Book Medical Publishers; 1970.

5. **Scura G, Davidoff F.** Case-related use of the medical literature: clinical librarian services for improving patient care. JAMA. 1981; 245:50-2.

6. **Marshall JG.** The impact of the hospital library on clinical decision-making: the Rochester study. Bull Med Libr Assoc. 1992;80:169-78.

7. **Klein MS, Ross FV, Adams DL, Gilbert CM.** Effect of on-line literature searching on length of stay and patient care costs. Acad Med. 1994;69:489-95.

8. **Purcell GP, Shortliffe EH.** Contextual models of clinical publications for enhancing retrieval from full-text databases. Nineteenth Annual Symposium on Computer Applications in Medical Care. October 28–November 1, 1995. New Orleans: McGraw-Hill; 1995: 851-7.

9. **Tierney WM, Miller ME, Overhage JM, McDonald CJ.** Physician inpatient order writing on microcomputer workstations. Effects on resource utilization. JAMA. 1993;269:379-83.

10. **McDonald CH, Hui SL, Smith DM, Tierney WM, Cohen SJ, Weinberger M, et al.** Reminders to physicians from an introspective computer medical record: a two-year randomized trial. Ann Intern Med. 1984;100:130-4.

11. **Berner ES, Webster GD, Shugerman AA, Jackson JR, Algina J, Baker AL.** Performance of four computer-based diagnostic systems. N Engl J Med. 1994;330:1824-5.

12. **Miller RA, Maserie FE Jr.** The demise of the Greek Oracle model for medical diagnostic systems. Meth Information Med. 1990;29:1-2.

CHAPTER 4

Is Basic Science Necessary?

S ome years ago, E.B. White and James Thurber wrote a book called *Is Sex Necessary?*, a title obviously intended to evoke a "You've got to be kidding" reaction among readers. The question "Is basic science necessary?" at first has something of the same impact, particularly when considered in the context of the teaching and the practice of clinical medicine. But important recent work by a number of educational scholars, in particular Schmidt and colleagues in Holland (1,2), is forcing us to recognize the seriousness of the question, and to examine more deeply many of our dearly held assumptions about the relationship between basic science and clinical medicine.

The question gains immediacy from the observation that computerized diagnostic support systems perform reasonably well compared with seasoned human diagnosticians (3), yet the information encoded in these systems consists virtually entirely of clinical knowledge and almost no basic science. (For the purposes of this discussion, following Schmidt, the term *basic science* is used interchangeably with *biomedical science* and *pathophysiologic knowledge*. All of these refer to the pathological principles, mechanisms, or processes underlying the manifestations of disease. In contrast, terms such as *clinical knowledge* and *clinical concepts* denote the ways in which a disease can manifest itself in patients, the kind of complaints one would expect, given that disease, the nature and variability of the signs and symptoms, and the ways in which the disease can be managed [2].)

The sharp discontinuity between the received wisdom that basic science is essential to clinical medicine and the lack of basic science in well-functioning electronic diagnostic systems parallels a widespread but rarely acknowledged experience of medical students, most of whom breathe at least a metaphoric sigh of relief when their basic science years in medical school are over. For at that point not only do they begin to learn the "real" clinical medicine they will later use every day in practice, but they are intrigued, albeit a bit puzzled, to discover that the clinical knowledge requisite to excellent clinical practice seems to draw on only a small fraction of what they've learned in their basic science courses. The recent and rather appalling finding that half of all students in medical schools with traditional curricula learn at least half of their basic science material by rote (which they defined by expressions like "engraving an equation, dictum, or passage from a textbook or lecture into my mind, repeating it over and over until I can spew it out on cue . . . not comprehending a word of it") confirms these subjective impressions, and certainly does not speak well for the enduring value of basic science to clinicians (4). Interestingly, only 6 percent of students in school using a problem-based learning curriculum felt they had learned 50 percent or more of their basic sciences by rote. In contrast, less than 10 percent of students in both traditional and problem-based schools felt they learned as much as half of their clinical material by rote.

The discontinuity between basic discipline and applied practice is hardly unique to medicine, however. After all, musicians learn to be superb performers without extensive formal knowledge of harmony or the rules of composition. Airline pilots become expert in flying without understanding the thermodynamics of jet engines. And children are fluent in language long before they learn explicit rules of grammar. Scholars interested in understanding the relationships between basic science and clinical medicine therefore have a good deal to chew on from studies of the development of expertise in other fields.

Schmidt and his colleagues (1,2) approached the problem in a very straightforward way. Subjects were asked to "think aloud" about their diagnostic reasoning, describe the underlying pathophysiology, or recall clinical details from memory in response to brief clinical cases presented to them in writing. Working from the written or audiotaped responses, the authors quantitatively characterized each statement, using detailed, formal analytic methods.

Their most startling finding, which confirmed and extended previous work, was that the most experienced clinicians used the least biomedical knowledge in understanding a case and arriving at a diagnosis (1). The authors concluded, first, that "the transition from the application of biomedical knowledge to the application of clinical knowledge seems to be associated with the transition from preclinical to clinical education," and, second, that this transition is "rather abrupt." Equally intriguing was their observation that "intermediate" medical students (roughly the equivalent of second year students in the United States) used the largest number of biomedical concepts in their diagnostic thinking (2), more than *either* beginning students *or* experienced clinicians. A graph of biomedical concept use plotted against experience thus revealed an inverted U-shaped curve, which the authors termed the "intermediate effect."

It seems easy enough to explain why "intermediate" students use more biomedical concepts than beginners; after all, basic science concepts are all they've been given to work with up to that point, along with a clear message that this basic science material is the very stuff that will allow them to practice the best scientific medicine. But how can it be that the experienced clinicians had moved away from using basic science? Were the experimental methods flawed? Were these clinicians, in fact, not competent or representative? The data, taken together with the careful experimental design, seem to rule out these other explanations and lead us directly to the counterintuitive conclusion that it is expert clinicians who actually use the least biomedical knowledge in dealing with clinical problems.

In more recent work, Schmidt's group (2) has addressed the question of why and how clinicians operate in this unexpected way. To do so, they tested three hypotheses about the structure of basic biomedical knowledge in expert clinicians' minds, namely that such knowledge is

1. Inert—forgotten, unretrievable, expunged;
2. Still there, but exists in a kind of parallel world, separate from clinical knowledge, hence rarely used; or
3. Still there, but encapsulated within, and closely linked to, clinical knowledge.

It is reassuring and, perhaps, not entirely surprising that the data of Schmidt and colleagues clearly support the third hypothesis. Moreover, they find that biomedical knowledge encapsulated in expert clinicians' minds exists in a shorthand form in which many small information "pixels" are aggregated or chunked together into larger, intermediate-level knowledge structures (e.g., "septic state" instead of "bacterial toxin stimulates cytokine release, leading to fever, sweats, rigors, flushed skin, tachycardia, hypotension"), making the summed information quickly and easily accessible.

An important related finding of these and other researchers is that expert clinicians presented with medical problems outside their main area of expertise "downshift" from using a few encapsulated pathophysiologic concepts to using many, detailed but more "primitive" pathophysiologic constructs (2). In the world of clinical practice, basic pathophysiologic knowledge thus appears to serve as a kind of intellectual safety net. This fallback mechanism allows clinicians who find themselves beyond their domain of expertise to reason their way in a respectable fashion through complex or unfamiliar problems by using first principles—situations in which their usual fluid use of clinical grammar has failed them and their clinical performance would otherwise degrade ungracefully.

Moreover, these "ontologic" shifts in the everyday diagnostic strategies of practicing clinicians seem to recapitulate the original "phylogenetic" evolution of the medical students as their diagnostic strategies mature. Thus, from the exhaustive (and exhausting!) assembly of "undigested" detail of their preclinical years, students progress to the use of hypothecodeductive reasoning, once they have acquired enough knowledge to generate and test diagnostic hypotheses (5); they then move on to an algorithmic approach (the "if-then" rules beloved of residents for dealing with the most common, most important, and most difficult clinical situations) and, finally, to the almost instant "gestalt" recognition of clinical states that characterizes the expert who has "seen it all" (Table 1).

Schmidt's observations could be interpreted to mean that clinicians can achieve an advanced level of expertise only by passing through the tradi-

TABLE 1
Use of basic science concepts in the diagnostic process:
relation to level of expertise

Level of Expertise	Use of Basic Science	Nature of Concepts Used	Dominant Diagnostic Strategy
Preclinical	Moderate	Detailed	Exhaustive
Clinical student	Most	Detailed	Hypotheco-deductive
Resident/ fellow	Substantial	Some encapsulated	Algorithmic
Expert clinician	Least	Encapsulated	Gestalt

tional sequence of stages: basic science, followed by clinical learning, and finally the encapsulation of basic science into clinical concepts. An alternative interpretation is also possible, however: that the traditional sequence is an accident of history rather than a fundamental law of nature; that basic science learning is not an essential precursor of, and may contribute only in limited ways to, the learning of clinical skill and performance.

It is possible to interpret these data to mean that basic science learning slows down clinical learning or may even interfere with it. In the latter case, students of medicine would be better off if they learned "in reverse," that is, first learning how to obtain and use clinical information, only then "dipping down" to obtain basic science knowledge, and doing so only to the depth needed to undergird their clinical thinking. (Could this, in fact, be a partial description of problem-based learning?)

As usual, new insights like these raise as many questions as they answer:

- Would clinicians trained "in reverse" function better within their areas of clinical expertise than those trained in the traditional fashion? Or would they be pseudoclinicians, practicing a kind of "cookbook" medicine that worked well as long as they didn't stray from familiar territory but that crashed whenever an unusual clinical problem came along?
- Would medicine become less scientific than it is now, and, if so, what would be the effect of that?
- Would the "reverse" approach represent a move toward anti-intellectualism, a kind of medical "cultural revolution"? Or would "reverse" training of clinicians break the current hold of basic science over medical training that many see as rigid and stifling?
- Would the "reverse" approach use precious student and faculty time more efficiently and effectively (6)?
- Does anyone, anywhere, have the courage, the resources, and the patience to set up a rigorous controlled trial of these two opposite approaches to medical training?
- And how, for heaven's sake, could a subject this important have been neglected for this long to begin with?

With studies like those of Schmidt and his colleagues, we appear finally to be gaining some real understanding of the role of basic science in the practice of clinical medicine, in contradistinction to its role in developing new tools to be used in the practice of medicine—the two are not at all the same. At the very least, the studies by these patient, thoughtful researchers teach us that we can't afford *not* to understand the real role of basic science in the learning and practicing of clinical medicine; that the best possible care ultimately depends on an honest and deep understanding of that role. Their work and that of others in this key area deserves strong continued support. We are very much in their debt.

REFERENCES

1. Boshuizen HA, Schmidt HG. On the role of biomedical knowledge in clinical reasoning by experts, intermediates and novices. Cognitive Science. 1992;16:153-84.
2. Schmidt HG, Norman GR, Boshuizen HA. On the origin of intermediate effects in clinical case recall. Mem Cognit. 1993;21:338-51.
3. Berner ES, Webster GD, Shugerman AA, Jackson JR, Algina J, Baker AL, et al. Performance of four computer-based diagnostic systems. N Engl J Med. 1994;330:1792-6.
4. Regan-Smith MG, Obenshain SS, Woodward C, Richards B, Zeitz HJ, Small DJ. Rote learning in medical school. JAMA. 1994; 272:1380-1.
5. Elstein AS, Shulman LS, Sprafka SA. Medical Problem Solving: An Analysis of Clinical Reasoning. Cambridge, MA: Harvard University Press; 1978.
6. Marston RQ, Jones RM, eds. Medical Education in Transition. Commission on Medical Education: The Sciences of Medical Practice. Princeton, NJ: Robert Wood Johnson Foundation; 1992.

CHAPTER 5

The Voytovich Solution

Mr. Kovacs is a 60-year-old coal miner who presents to your office with a five-year history of increasing dyspnea. He drinks four to five beers per day and a quart of whiskey per week, mostly on weekends. He now has experienced 2 to 3 days of malaise, fever, chills, and increasing amounts of rusty, purulent sputum. On physical examination you find a blood pressure of 170/100, a pulse of 120 beats per minute and regular, and a temperature of 39° C orally. Fundi show marked arterial narrowing and arteriovenous compression. There are rales, dullness, egophony, and increased tactile fremitus over the left upper lung field posteriorly. The liver is felt 5 cm below the right costal margin and is slightly tender; the rest of the examination is unremarkable.

The patient's laboratory results include the following: Hct = 40, WBC = 16,000 with 60 polys, 18 bands, 12 lymphs, 8 monos, 2 eos. A Gram stain of his sputum is loaded with polys and gram-positive diplococci. Chest film shows a dense lobar infiltrate in the left upper lobe. Blood culture obtained the night before is growing *Streptococcus pneumoniae*.

*M*r. Kovacs is not an unusual patient for a busy internist; his problems are not excessively complex. But he certainly is a "multiproblem" patient, that is, several things are going on medically at the same time. What's more, because his particular combination of problems is unique, you won't find a patient exactly like him in any medical textbook.

Multiproblem patients are a challenge to medicine. They are a particular challenge to general internists, who more frequently than other specialists are asked to sort out the diagnostic complexities and manage the interacting comorbidities of multiple organ systems—not to mention dysfunctional psychosocial systems as well. But how is it possible to organize the complex information in Mr. Kovacs' case? What is the best way to express what's going on with him? How could you find out how well a student, a resident, or a colleague has understood his many problems? And how in the world would you teach someone else to understand them?

The work of Anthony Voytovich provides powerful insights for understanding as well as tools for managing, teaching, and learning about these crucial, albeit subtle and demanding, tasks. Unfortunately, the enormous sophistication and utility of this work are not yet widely recognized or used to their full advantage. Dr. Voytovich, who spent his formative years with Thomas Hale Ham and Lawrence Weed at Case Western Reserve University and who is now professor of medicine at the University of Connecticut Health Center in Farmington, describes sorting out the clinical clues presented by patients like Mr. Kovacs as being like sorting a pile of jigsaw puzzle pieces and assembling the puzzle. But this is not an ordinary puzzle-doer's task; there are several additional "zingers" in the situation since 1) there may be more than one puzzle, 2) any one or all of the puzzles may be incomplete, 3) some pieces fit more than one of the puzzles, and 4) some pieces don't fit any of the puzzles (1). In a nutshell (to paraphrase Bette Davis's comment about aging): Clinical reasoning about multiproblem patients is not for sissies.

How, then, to manage efficiently and reliably the information from multiproblem patients, information of almost Talmudic complexity? Voytovich makes a convincing case that there is a single organizing framework or instrument for putting it all together, that is, the Master Problem List—that innocent-looking assemblage of items usually found in the front of the patient's chart but all too often underused or ignored. At the same time, Voytovich makes the case that the huge potential of the problem list can only be realized if it is used right, that is, according to certain very specific and rather strict rules. Handled this way, however, the problem list becomes an enormously powerful tool for clinical care, quality review, and teaching.

There is an elegant simplicity to Voytovich's basic rules for creating a high-quality problem list. First, the problem list has to be *complete;* that is, it must contain all items that are of concern to or require action by the patient and his or her physician. Second, the problem list has to be *precise;* that is, every problem on the list must be formulated (i.e., conceptualized and expressed) at exactly the level permitted by the available data, neither higher nor lower. At first, this all sounds rather fussy and pedantic. But Voytovich points out that the process of formulating a good problem list is no more obscure or extreme than balancing your checkbook: you can't leave out any entries, and all the arithmetic has to check out. And the penalty for not sticking to the rules is the same for both: you can find yourself in deep trouble in a hurry because you can't tell where you are.

At a deeper level, a properly constructed problem list is neither more nor less than a representation of the patient's medical concerns according to the Golden Rule: it does unto the patient what we would have done unto ourselves if we were sick. After all, who among us would like the summary of problems in our medical records to be incomplete, vague, sloppy, disorganized, inaccurate—like all too many existing master problem lists? A well-formulated problem list may, in fact, be one of the best expressions of truly "holistic" medicine, more so than most other formulations of that much abused concept.

But a complete, precise problem list is just the beginning. Once you have accepted the basic rules, you can then define a number of basic types of errors in problem formulation. This, in turn, allows you to decide whether any given problem list is or is not complete and precise, making it possible to create better problem lists, and hence to deliver better care. This also puts you in a very strong position to audit the quality of problem lists and to teach the essentials of clinical reasoning.

Most of the work by Voytovich and his colleagues over the past 15 years has been devoted to defining these basic errors and, using these definitions, to developing quantitative measures of problem list quality—in effect, a scoring system (2–5). Their extensive effort has revealed the existence of four, and only four, kinds of errors:

1. *Omission.* Omission means that an important clinical clue has simply been ignored. For example, proteinuria appears in the urinalysis report but is not included on the problem list.

2. *Premature closure.* This is a jumping to conclusions, that is, diagnostic formulation at a level not justified by the existing data. For example, the presence of both "anemia" and "rectal bleeding" is assumed to make a diagnosis of "iron deficiency."

3. *Inadequate synthesis.* This is more or less the opposite error: a level of diagnostic formulation is staring you in the face but is not recognized or accepted. For example, a history of typical anginal chest discomfort plus demonstration of 85 percent occlusion of the left main coronary artery on angiography are formulated only as "heart disease."

4. *Wrong formulations.* These are problem statements that are actually contradicted by the data. For example, "trace ketonuria" and "arterial pH = 7.42" are interpreted as "diabetic ketoacidosis."

Nonphysicians can be trained without much difficulty to "score" problem lists from both standardized cases (like that of Mr. Kovacs) (2) and real patient charts with high reliability (1). Using these techniques, Voytovich and his colleagues have described the frequency and behavior of each error type. Thus, they have found that omission occurs more frequently than the other three error types, whereas wrong formulations occur least frequently; the frequency of premature closures and of inadequate syntheses lies between these two extremes. Importantly, overall problem list scores distinguish reliably among second, third, and fourth year medical students and house officers (2), a more than respectable power of discrimination for a clinical evaluation instrument. With the use of a computer, it is also possible to score free-entry problem formulations and obtain results that resemble those obtained by hand scoring (6).

But most interesting of all, each type of error behaves distinctively. Thus, incomplete synthesis and omission correlate with training level; the tendency to make these two errors varies independently, but the tendency to make each one is consistent within individuals (7). Premature closure, in contrast, is found with equal frequency at all levels of training and clinical experience, and correlates with an independent measure of confidence (i.e., overconfidence) in knowledge relevant to the case at hand, but not to the overall level of medical knowledge. Both premature closure and inadequate synthesis also reflect physicians' estimates of disease likelihood which, in turn, are a component of the iterative and semiquantitative approach to clinical thinking known as "Bayesian reasoning" (8). Interestingly enough, however, these two errors behave differently in that premature closures are expressed in a uniform way, while there are at least four different expressions of inadequate synthesis (6).

It is sobering to consider the consequences of these errors. The effects of omission and wrong synthesis are self-evident. Inadequate synthesis is probably a major reason for unnecessary testing and delays in treatment, with their attendant implications of patient risk and excess resource consumption. In contrast, premature closure may defer appropriate testing and workup, delay or mask the correct diagnosis, and generate inappropriate treatment (5). (See Chapter 22, Confidence Testing.)

At the same time, the availability of validated techniques for formulating problems accurately and for identifying and quantifying errors in problem formulation is cause for celebration. To quote Voytovich, the scoreable problem list won't practice better medicine for you, any more than a mirror will make you beautiful. But, like the mirror, it can show you exactly where the deficiencies are, which is an enormous help if you are going to deliver the best possible care, particularly to multiproblem patients. Creating, analyzing, and scoring problem lists can certainly help you to know whether optimal care is being delivered, and to teach students and residents how to deliver it.

REFERENCES

1. **Voytovich AE, Harper L, Rippey RM.** Evaluating analytic reasoning in the management of the multiproblem patient: a system for attaining reliability and validity. Presented at the Conference on Research in Medical Education (RIME), Association of American Medical Colleges; 1979.
2. **Voytovich AE, Rippey RM, Copertino L.** Scoreable problem lists as measures of clinical judgment. Evaluation and Health Professions. 1980;3:159-70.
3. **Voytovich AE, Rippey RM.** Knowledge, realism, and diagnostic reasoning in a physical diagnosis course. J Med Educ. 1982;57:461-7.
4. **Voytovich AE, Rippey RM, Suffredini A.** Premature conclusions in diagnostic reasoning. J Med Educ. 1985;60:302-7.
5. **Dubeau CE, Voytovich AE, Rippey RM.** Premature conclusions in the diagnosis of iron-deficiency anemia: cause and effect. Med Decis Making. 1986;6:169-73.
6. **Voytovich AE, Rippey RM, Jue D.** Diagnostic reasoning in the multiproblem patient: an interactive, microcomputer audit. Evaluation and Health Professions. 1986;9:91-102.
7. **Voytovich AE, Rippey RM.** Audit of the structured problem list as a measure of clinical judgment: reliability and validity. Irish Med J. 1978;71:346-9.
8. **Thornton JG, Lilford RJ, Johnson N.** Decision analysis in medicine. BMJ. 1992;304:1099-103.

CHAPTER 6

Commitment for Change

⌒

A "Radioimmunoassay" for Continuing Medical Education

[with Kathleen L. Egan, PhD]

What would it be like to practice endocrinology without the radioimmunoassay? "Unthinkable," most endocrinologists would say today. But some of us are old enough to remember when only a few hormone assays were available, and those were crude: insensitive, nonspecific, expensive, slow, tedious. Then along came the radioimmunoassay: exquisitely sensitive, elegantly specific, relatively quick, and cheap. The rest, as they say, is history.

Continuing medical education (CME) isn't endocrinology. But to the extent that all disciplines share common challenges in measuring the effects of their interventions, CME might be said to be in its "pre-immunoassay" era.

Obviously, what CME outcomes we choose to measure will depend on what we believe is CME's real payoff. Is the principal intent to have participants achieve stated learning objectives? Acquire new knowledge? (These two are not necessarily the same.) Identify outmoded knowledge that should be dropped? Increase their confidence in valid knowledge? While all of these matter, most people would agree that they are inter-mediates, related only indirectly to the gold standard for CME, which is to improve patient outcomes.

But patient outcomes are hard to measure, so present-day CME programs rely largely on assays of those intermediates for which handy measures exist. A "happiness" index (Were you satisfied with the program?) is almost always included, and, occasionally, the assay extends to

29

some measure of knowledge retention, mostly in the form of multiple-choice questions.

It would be unrealistic, of course, to expect every part of every CME program to improve medical outcomes among every participant's patients. And most CME programs, particularly live events, also serve important social and professional purposes other than "pure" education. CME programs can, for instance, enhance participants' sense of professional identity, connect them with colleagues, and reassure them that their practices fall within some reasonable bound of variation, among other things, all of which must be considered important parts of professional life. On the other hand, if CME programs don't also change medical outcomes, why bother with them at all? Logically, therefore, we would expect a sensitive and specific assay for CME's effects to measure *change,* ideally in patient outcomes, or, failing that, at least to measure changes in clinical practices that are likely to result in improved outcomes. Enter the "commitment for change" strategy.

Introduced into CME circles several years ago (1), the commitment for change approach has much to recommend it. First, it's simple: At the end of each segment of a CME program, participants are asked to commit themselves in writing to one or more changes they intend to make in their practices, based on those points in the program they felt were sufficiently important, convincing, and relevant to their own practices.

Second, the commitment for change approach deals with explicit (observable) outcomes—actual changes in clinical practice—rather than implicit ones, such as changes in knowledge. The usual CME learning objectives are defined in terms of acquired knowledge. But at the same time, CME program directors are well aware that it is not enough to assume knowledge has actually been transferred from faculty to participants. As a consequence, they are forced to use action expressions like "will be able to explain," and the like to describe learning objectives, artfully chosen to make changes in the obscure and subtle internal state called "knowledge" into something explicit and observable. At the same time, directors are in the irrational and uncomfortable position of having to avoid accurate but non-documentable descriptions of learning outcomes like "will understand." Despite the careful crafting of these labored descriptions, however, participants are rarely asked at the end of a CME program to demonstrate that they are, in fact, "able to explain" their new understandings, and if they were asked, there would be no way to judge the adequacy of the explanations they produced. The commitment for change avoids all that.

Third, the commitment for change also avoids the cueing problem. Multiple-choice questions give away a lot. Choice of question content alone tells participants what the faculty considers most important. While this can help drive home key messages, it also draws attention away from other potentially important elements of the program. And since even modest-sized CME programs contain dozens, if not hundreds, of content elements, it is almost impossible for faculty to know a priori what learners may find most important for themselves and their practices. Stated differently, the content of the questions expresses the faculty's priorities, whether or not those are relevant to the learners' needs. And anyone who has gotten through medical school and residency knows how to use the structure of a multiple-choice question to help answer it. Answering a question correctly, therefore, doesn't always mean you really understand the topic.

The commitment for change approach, by contrast, is open-ended: It's up to the participants to make up their own minds about what's important, to actively filter out key issues from the program material (which seems an appropriate expectation of skilled professionals) rather than passively accepting the faculty's prescription. And the commitment for change short-circuits altogether the figuring out of answers from question structure.

Fourth, as an extension of the commitment for change process, faculty can write down beforehand the changes they would most like learners to implement in their practices as a result of their teaching. By comparing the commitments that participants write down at the end of the program to the faculty's a priori written expectations, it should then be possible to find out whether the two are even close. This fundamental question about CME has never been answered, partly, perhaps, because there was previously no other assay that could be used to answer it. The match (or mismatch, as the case may be) between faculty expectation and learner outcome measured in this way then becomes a tool for increasing the effectiveness of CME programs.

Fifth, the evaluation process used in the commitment for change approach may itself be a force for change. The psychological and management literature (2) makes it very clear that the very act of articulating and writing down behaviors you plan to change increases the likelihood that you'll actually change them (what in other settings is called "goal setting"). This self-reinforcing property of the commitment for change strategy may be one of its more important features, and it deserves more serious exploration in its own right.

Finally, and perhaps most importantly, weeks or months after a CME program, participants can be presented with the commitments they wrote down earlier and asked if they have implemented the changes. The frequency of change thus becomes a direct measure of CME program effectiveness, and while it falls short of the measurement of patient outcomes, it is closer to that gold standard than expressions of global satisfaction with a CME course, or facts remembered. Participants who report they have not made the changes can then be asked why they haven't. Their reasons (which may of course include absence of encounters with the appropriate patients and lack of support services, equipment, or other necessary resources) provide additional insights into the process by which CME actually translates into practice.

Of course, the commitment for change strategy is not without its problems. Data collection is labor-intensive and fairly expensive. Without considerable guidance, participants tend to express their commitments in language too vague or abstract to be useful—for example, "I intend to be more aware of [problem] . . ." Analysis of written commitments requires appropriate taxonomic clusters or groupings, but techniques for creating them are not easy or widely understood. The response rate to the follow-up on implementation in practice is often low. And, of course, reports of implementation depend on the subjective judgments of participant physicians, which raises questions about the reliability and validity of the data.

These problems notwithstanding, the commitment for change strategy promises to be a useful innovation, particularly in CME programs where the outcomes are so concrete. And although there are clearly problems to be overcome, most of them should be manageable, given enough time and effort. The accuracy of self-reporting of practice implementation, for example, could be established by the appropriate studies using chart audits or patient interviews; and it also should be possible to develop efficient techniques for collecting, abstracting, and summarizing physicians' written commitments. The radioimmunoassay, after all, is also complex and technically demanding and was not perfected in a day.

While the radioimmunoassay was purely a technological advance, its power was such that it transformed medicine in fundamental ways, which is why its designers received the Nobel Prize. The commitment for change strategy may not transform CME as dramatically, but refocusing and sharpening our assays may provide an important link that is now missing from the overall CME process. And CME these days, like medicine itself, needs all the help it can get.

REFERENCES

1. **Jones D.** Viability of the commitment for change evaluation strategy. In: Research in Medical Education. Proceedings of the 29th Annual Conference sponsored by the Association of American Medical Colleges. October 1990; San Francisco. Acad Med. 1990;65(9 Suppl):S37-8.
2. **Locke ED, Shaw KN, Saari LM, Latham GP.** Goal setting and task performance: 1969–1980. Psychol Bull. 1981;91:125-52.

CHAPTER 7

Lifelong Learning

C ontinuous self-improvement, a.k.a. lifelong learning or continuing scholarship, is a hallmark of all true professionalism. Idealistic but vague pronouncements on the importance of lifelong learning recur throughout medical school and residency, and the exhortations continue on out into the practice years. Curiously, however, for a principle held in such high regard, the Special Requirements that govern internal medicine residencies are vague on the topic, mentioning only that residents should maintain "a commitment to scholarship . . . and . . . to continued improvement," but providing no clue as to how to go about doing so (1). And, paradoxically, the exhortations become more muted during the practice years, precisely the part of one's career when they should be loudest and most forceful.

Despite its righteous purpose, precious little is known or taught anywhere in medicine about lifelong learning. And particularly when it comes to facing up to the hard realities of maintaining lifelong learning in the context of a busy practice—the secrets of learning on a continuing and lifelong basis—there is considerably more rhetoric than realization, more lip service than performance.

Medical school and residency themselves are, of course, specifically designed to create rich learning environments for those who live in them. Life during these years is structured so that learners' principal responsibility—in fact, their professional survival—lies above all in learning, rather than in the delivery of patient care. Concern for lifelong learning extends only about as far as the expression of hope that, despite the virtual absence of explicit, practical attention to the subject, at least some learning about *how* to learn during the rest of a career will rub off on students and residents.

But on the day they leave residency, newly minted physicians step out of the protected world of education into the demanding, turbulent world of practice, where professional survival (not to mention patient survival) lies principally in the delivery of high-quality medical care, not in learning. Or, more precisely, active, formal learning inevitably gets pushed into the background among the rigors of patient responsibility and the pressure of daily clinical work; the effort to learn on a continuing basis thus becomes a never-ending struggle more than a daily imperative.

Standard, lecture-type continuing medical education (CME) recreates in microcosm some of the learning environment of the initial years of training, and as such can help in the struggle to keep on learning. But practicing doctors participate only intermittently in formal CME, and formal CME, by itself, is only modestly and transiently effective in changing medical knowledge and practice (2). So it is good news that at least a few serious efforts are being made to move the state of the art of lifelong learning beyond traditional CME. There is now, for example, some experience with tailored learning programs (3). David Sackett and his colleagues at McMaster University (4) have given a great deal of thought to the techniques of keeping up to date and have shared their experience with methods for reviewing one's own performance, tracking down evidence, choosing journals to read, surveying the medical literature, critically appraising articles, and the like. Then there are a variety of self-assessment instruments such as the American College of Physicians' Medical Knowledge Self-Assessment Program (MKSAP) specifically designed to support physicians in their efforts to evaluate the state of their own knowledge, and teach themselves. (See Chapter 11, Mirror, Mirror.) And now, of course, specialty board recertification provides added impetus for all this effort.

The bad news is that, despite all the work and creativity that have gone into them, these special programs are extremely labor-intensive, and their use remains the exception rather than the rule. We are still far from having thought through the matter of lifelong learning as thoroughly as it deserves; in sum, we lack a "deep" solution to the problem. To be sure, it would be unrealistic to look for a magic bullet, a single-shot solution to the problem of lifelong learning. However, it is not too much to expect that we can achieve a more profound understanding of lifelong learning, the kind that is needed for an elegant, inexpensive, effective, and efficient solution; a true high echnology, in contrast to the existing clumsy, expensive, half-way technology; a polio vaccine rather than an iron lung (5).

Enter David Seegal. Seegal was on the clinical faculty at Columbia University's College of Physicians and Surgeons some decades ago. He taught us medicine at the Goldwater Hospital, a vast realm of chronic disease on an island in New York City's East River. In that unlikely setting, we learned not only about exciting and important clinical things, like valvular heart disease and dermatology, but also important pedagogical things, like *how* to learn—ideas and principles that resonate in his students to this day.

The first of Seegal's memorable teachings about lifelong learning came at the end of our long afternoons with patients when he asked each of us: "Well, what did you learn today?" Thinking back on it, this deceptively simple question clearly embodies the deep principle of *reflection,* later elaborated by Donald Schön in his concept of *reflective practitioner* (6). In his quiet way, then, and without our being aware of it, Seegal brought us to the realization that lifelong learning requires a particular state of mind—a receptive, reflective state—as much as it requires a particular skill or technique. Reflection, in this sense, means asking yourself (as often as possible) "What were the 'take-homes' from that reading, or from that consultation, or from that patient, or from that clinical experience?"—and then going out and tracking down the answer to the question. The idea of reflection expresses the difference between learning as simply taking in information and learning in the deeper sense of *metanoia* (from the Greek roots *meta-,* above or beyond; and *noia,* from the root *nous,* mind), that is, bringing about a fundamental shift or movement of mind—a change in mental models (7).

Seegal's second teaching about lifelong learning was expressed in the mysterious formula he wrote on the blackboard early in our rotation at Goldwater:

$$WD_{LB} + LU_{BB} = K$$

Translated, this turned out to mean: If you Write it Down in the Little Book, then Look it Up in the Big Book, your Knowledge will grow. The "it," of course, referred to anything you had seen or heard in the course of working with patients that you hadn't understood. The Little Book was any place one might keep *written* notes and reminders where they wouldn't get lost or mixed up; nowadays, of course, this might be a palmtop computer. The Big Book back then was mostly Cecil and Loeb's textbook (Robert Loeb was still Chair of Medicine at Columbia!); now, of course, it would include a whole universe of print and electronic information sources.

Seegal had again captured in his concise way a number of key principles, ideas that would later emerge as part of two important formal educational perspectives: 1) adult learning—that is, active, case-related inquiry based on the need to know, accompanied by prompt feedback and reinforcement (8); and 2) experiential learning—that is, participation in real experience, which is then linked to reflection on what happened (problem formulation), development of a conceptual framework that explains and guides action, and, finally, experimentation with new and better ways of dealing with experience (9). (See Chapter 24, The Right Hand of Claude.) But Seegal had, in addition, adapted these principles into a convenient and flexible form, so they might actually work in the life of a busy student—or throughout the life of a busy clinical practitioner. It would be hard to imagine a simpler or more effective, nuts-and-bolts technique to support the reflective state of mind.

For all its elegant simplicity and conceptual power, Seegal's learning legacy was until recently shared primarily among those few who were lucky enough to study with him. And, interestingly, the entire formal CME system in the United States seems to have been built on principles that are virtually antithetical to that legacy. (See Chapter 30, Does Continuing Medical Education Work?) But deep understandings have a way of not remaining hidden. Thus it is that former students of David Seegal will be pleased to learn about the Maintenance of Competence Program (MOCOMP), the system recently introduced in Canada by their Royal College of Physicians and Surgeons to support lifelong learning in that country. For while Seegal's teachings themselves did not directly influence its creation, the MOCOMP system clearly embodies both the reflective frame of mind and the Little Book approach (10).

Under this innovative plan, Canadian physicians are asked literally to write down, day in, day out, their clinical questions (the MOCOMP initially provided a paper booklet for this purpose, but later shifted to an electronic recording system). Participating physicians are also asked to say where these questions came from (e.g., patient, conference, reading, colleague) and to describe the outcome of their learning efforts (e.g., new understanding, change in practice, need for more information)—in effect, what "fundamental shifts of mind" occur as they look for answers in the Big Book(s). And, finally, CME credit is awarded for this effort: for units of *learning*, rather than for hours spent as participants in organized, fee-based CME programs (or, in other words, for units of *exposure to teaching*). This seems only rational since, as the designers of the MOCOMP point out, the amount learned correlates poorly with the amount of time spent being taught. (However, the MOCOMP does also encourage participation in organized CME programs.) (See Chapter 37, Units of Learning, Not Units of Teaching.)

Only time will tell how well MOCOMP will work in Canada—the initial experience has been positive (11)—and whether its principles will spread southward across the border and elsewhere in the world. But it does contain many important and attractive features (see Chapter 37, Units of Learning, Not Units of Teaching and Chapter 6, Commitment for Change) that support true self-determined growth, or what is now referred to in some quarters as "continuing professional development," to distinguish it from more traditional continuing medical education. How gratifying to know that David Seegal lives. It encourages us to believe that lifelong learning lives along with him.

REFERENCES

1. **Accreditation Council for Graduate Medical Education.** Revised Special Requirements for Residency Training Programs in Internal Medicine. Graduate Medical Education Directory. Chicago: American Medical Association; 1993.
2. **Davis DA, Thomson MA, Oxman AD, Haynes RB.** Changing physician performance. A systematic review of the effect of continuing medical education strategies. JAMA. 1995;274:700-5.
3. **Manning PR, Clintworth WA, Sinopoli LM, Taylor JP, Krochalk PC, Gilman NJ.** A method of self-directed learning in continuing medical education with implications for recertification. Ann Intern Med. 1989;107:909-13.
4. **Sackett DL, Haynes R, Guyatt GH, Tugwell P.** Clinical Epidemiology: A Basic Science for Clinical Medicine. 2nd ed. Boston: Little, Brown; 1991.
5. **Thomas L.** The technology of medicine. In: The Lives of a Cell: Notes of a Biology Watcher. New York: Viking Press; 1974:31-6.
6. **Schön D.** Educating the Reflective Practitioner: Toward a New Design for Teaching and Learning in the Professions. San Francisco: Jossey-Bass; 1988.
7. **Senge P.** The Fifth Discipline. The Art and Practice of the Learning Organization. New York: Doubleday; 1990.
8. **Knowles MS.** The Modern Practice of Adult Education. Chicago: AP Follett; 1980.

9. **Kolb DA.** Experiential Learning. Experience as the Source of Learning and Development. Englewood Cliffs, NJ: PTR Prentice Hall; 1984.

10. **Royal College of Physicians and Surgeons of Canada.** The maintenance of competence program. Ann Roy Coll Phys Surg Canada. 1993;26(Suppl):S3-53.

11. **Evans I.** Canada's style of continuing medical education. Lancet. 1995;346:1093.

CHAPTER 8

The Gold Standard of Evidence

❧

Archie Cochrane and Systematic Reviews

*A*s a clinician, how often have you had trouble deciding whether to use a particular diagnostic or therapeutic intervention, even one you were familiar with, because you were uncertain about how well it worked—or even whether it worked at all? Think how you've been frustrated by the difficulty of finding published studies on certain medical topics, and those few you did find only after wading through a small mountain of irrelevant references. Recall how many of the relevant studies turned out to be poorly done, how even the better studies were inconclusive, how bewildering it was to find inconsistent results across studies, some showing significant effects in one direction, some in the opposite direction, others showing no effect at all.

Or reflect on how often a colleague—or a resident, a student, or a drug detail person—has handed you (or quoted) an article that made a case for (or against) an important medical point when your own understanding of the literature didn't jibe with the proffered reference. How often have you had, in effect, the impression that, while such a reference was the truth, it wasn't the whole truth; that if you could only have gotten your hands on the whole truth, quickly and easily, a clinical decision would have been different?

The literal, ultimate "whole truth" on a given medical intervention is, of course, unknowable. But most clinicians, being pragmatic in such matters, would gladly settle for the next best thing, namely, access to the best evidence available in the world, the gold standard of evidence. The idea of a gold standard of evidence is intriguing, and while it now seems an obvious concept, it has not always been so. Indeed, it was only a decade ago that scholars like Diamond and Forrester began asking the really tough, ultimate "questions about questions" (or, in their terms, "meta-questions") about medical information (1). In the course of their work, these authors eventually arrived at the meta-question of "How much information is in any real information system?" (e.g., your head, textbooks, files, local practice community) relative to the total amount of information potentially available anywhere in the world—that is, relative to the gold standard. Their answer was that the information content of a real information system could be defined and measured in terms of its "orderliness"—in other words, how well that system provides access to the total information available anywhere (i.e., the gold standard). Lack of order, or "entropy," then is a measure of the degree to which a real system falls short of attaining the gold standard.

Diamond and Forrester graphically illustrated the concept of entropy by describing a library (a type of local information gold standard) in which much of the total information it contains is unavailable to users because cards are missing from the card catalogue or because the librarians have been reshelving volumes at random. In brief, the information is there; you just can't get at it because disorder—entropy—prevents you from doing so. The situation in medicine as a whole is somewhat more complicated, since it is estimated that high-quality or sound evidence exists anywhere in the world for only slightly more than half of what we do clinically (2). Even more startling is the estimate that only about 40 percent of this sound evidence demonstrates effectiveness, while 60 percent of it is evidence for the *lack* of value of current clinical interventions (3). But the imperfect nature of the existing gold standard aside, the sad truth is that in the real world it is very hard for most clinicians to get their hands on the evidence, including the highest quality evidence, that does exist. That information is widely scattered, not clearly marked, difficult to retrieve, not filtered on the basis of quality—all of which, in Diamond and Forrester's terms, means that the entropy of the entire medical information system is very high.

Jump ahead, now, to the year 2025. You are confronted with yet another vexingly uncertain clinical situation, much like the ones mentioned at the beginning of this chapter. This time, however, you simply turn to your handy electronic information device (the successor to the computer) and pull up an index of all the diagnostic and therapeutic maneuvers in medicine and their associated effects on clinical outcomes. Pointing to the intervention and outcome you're interested in, you are instantly presented with an up-to-date (and dated) "systematic review," a narrative and tables summarizing the findings from all known well-conducted randomized controlled trials, plus other appropriate evidence of similarly high quality—that is, data that meet certain clearly specified design criteria. You then jump down to another level in your information device where you can look at the original data extracted from these trials. You then inspect a formal synthesis (meta-analysis) of these data that includes a point estimate of the intervention's effect derived from the combined studies, along with the associated confidence intervals. These meta-analyses are neatly displayed in a graphic format that allows the data largely to speak for themselves (4). And looking at this information, it becomes obvious that when the results of many smaller studies are combined, the aggregate evidence is frequently conclusive, even though no single study can make that claim.

The good news is that if you are an obstetrician, this futuristic scenario is already a reality (5), created primarily through a rapidly developing movement in medical information systems called the Cochrane Collaboration (6). The bad news is that systematic reviews are for the most part available only in obstetrics and neonatal medicine, although more are appearing all the time in other medical disciplines now that the techniques for preparing them have been developed and are becoming more widely known (7). (These reviews are available in a variety of electronic formats, including floppy disks, CDs, and, increasingly, on the World Wide Web.) The movement takes its name from Archie Cochrane, who directed the South Wales Epidemiology Unit of the Medical Research Council in Great Britain in the 1960s and 1970s. Cochrane became an early and eloquent exponent of the use of high-quality evidence in medicine; he particularly championed the randomized controlled trial as the fundamental building block of such evidence; he helped carry out a number of important clinical trials. His Rock Carling Lecture entitled "Effectiveness and Efficiency: Random Reflections on Health Services," later published as a book, established him as one of the clearest and most influential thinkers in modern clinical epidemiology.

Cochrane was acutely aware of the disorder (high entropy) in the medical information system generally, and worked tirelessly to reduce it. In fact, the Collaboration was launched largely in response to his comment, now widely quoted, that "it is surely a great criticism of our profession that we have not *organized* a critical summary, by specialty or subspecialty, adapted periodically, of all relevant randomized controlled trials" (emphasis added). The mission of the Collaboration is to overcome that criticism through "preparing, maintaining, and disseminating systematic reviews of the effects of health care" (6).

Preparing systematic reviews is analogous to putting the cards back (in the right order!) into a library's card catalogue: a way of increasing the "orderliness" in the total medical information system. The rationale and steps in this process, as well as some of its potential pitfalls, have been well described recently (7). The first requirement in preparing a systematic review and perhaps the most important one, since it is aimed closest to the heart of the system's disorder, is to conduct an exhaustive search to *identify* all randomized controlled trials in a given clinical area. The search needs to include both published and unpublished trials, since only about 50 to 75 percent of all well-conducted randomized controlled trials are eventually published. Carrying out such a search may be a daunting task, but it is one that is actually beginning to seem manageable (8). (The recent decision by the National Library of Medicine to create the Medical Subject Heading [MeSH] terms "Controlled Clinical Trial" and "Randomized Controlled Trial" and, with the help of the medical journals, to identify and tag, both retrospectively and prospectively, all controlled trials in the MEDLINE database is an important step in supporting the production of systematic reviews.)

Defining the aim of the review, specifying the criteria for selecting trials, extracting and combining the data, presenting, interpreting, and, ultimately, disseminating the results are all part of the Cochrane process. The intent, and the hope, of the Cochrane Collaboration is that, over time, continuously updated systematic reviews will be prepared and made available in all areas of medicine (mainly in electronic form, which will allow timely critique and revision of reviews as new high-quality evidence becomes available), an "entropy-reducing" vision of staggering proportions but one which, as noted above, is actually beginning to happen.

Certainly, there is more to clinical medicine than having access to gold standard information (3), and learning clinical medicine involves a good deal more than knowing that such a gold standard exists and knowing how to use it (9). But in the greater scheme of things, it is arguably more important for all who practice medicine to learn about the quality of evidence and how close their own knowledge is to a gold standard than about the many other things they are now required to learn.

In educational circles, there is a saying that "if you want to learn about something, read about it. If you want to learn it better, teach it to someone. And if you want to learn it better still, program it into a computer." In a similar vein, the best way for students and residents (and the rest of us) to learn about the quality of evidence and the information gold standard might be for them (and us) to create a systematic review. Creating a systematic review is of necessity a group undertaking. Using the Cochrane group process as a model, students and residents who produced a systematic review would therefore come to appreciate, among other things, the realities and the rewards of this intense collaborative work.

Production of each review would require careful supervision by knowledgeable and committed faculty, but the process would create a close, working bond between faculty and students. It would cost little except time, and would require little in the way of tangible resources besides a good library, some well-trained librarians, electronic literature-searching capabilities, some microcomputers, some pencils, and paper. For the most part, what it would require is clear, orderly thinking, organization, and enthusiasm. And best of all, it would produce useful work: real, live systematic reviews that could (once they had passed through the appropriate editorial review) become part of the growing body of gold standard information.

Thus constituted, student and resident systematic review groups might ultimately become an important arm of the Cochrane Collaboration itself, helping it to build on itself by preparing both the contributors and the users of gold standard information of the future. Archie Cochrane would have liked the idea.

REFERENCES

1. **Diamond G, Forrester JS.** Metadiagnosis. An epistemologic model of clinical judgment. Am J Med. 1983;75:129-37.
2. **Ellis J, Mulligan I, Rowe J, Sackett DL.** Inpatient general medicine is evidence based. A-team, Nuffield Department of Clinical Medicine. Lancet. 1995;346:407-10.
3. **Haynes RB.** Some problems in applying evidence in clinical practice. Ann N Y Acad Sci. 1993;703:210-24.
4. **Goodman SN, Berlin JA.** The use of predicted confidence intervals when planning experiments and the misuse of power when interpreting results. Ann Intern Med. 1994;121:200-6.

5. **Chalmers I, Enkin M, Keirse MC, eds.** Effective Care in Pregnancy and Childbirth. Vols. 1 and 2. New York: Oxford University Press; 1991.
6. **Chalmers I.** The Cochrane Collaboration: preparing, maintaining, and disseminating systematic reviews of the effects of health care. Ann N Y Acad Sci. 1993;703:156-63.
7. **Chalmers I, Altman DG, eds.** Systematic Reviews. London: BMJ Publishing Group; 1995.
8. **Dickersin K, Scherer R, Lefebvre C.** Identifying relevant studies for systematic reviews. BMJ. 1994;309:1286-91.
9. **Lomas J.** Diffusion, dissemination, and implementation: who should do what? Ann N Y Acad Sci. 1993;703:226-35.

CHAPTER 9

Curriculum Is the Answer.
What Is the Question?

Curriculum is in the air. No matter what the problem in medical education, curriculum is looked to as the solution. Curriculum committees abound. Conferences on curriculum sprout like mushrooms. Journal supplements devoted to curriculum pour from the presses. The varieties of curriculum are many: Generalist Curriculum; Geriatrics Curriculum; Curriculum for Retraining Specialists; Community-Based Curriculum . . . the list goes on.

Even the normally staid Residency Review Committee in Internal Medicine has caught curriculum fever. More exactly, the Special Requirements (the detailed written standards by which residency programs are judged) that went into effect on July 1, 1994 required something they had never required before: "The structure of the program, including both patient-based and didactic elements, must be set down in a concise written document (in effect, a curriculum)" (1).

Beleaguered residency program directors are concerned that these new requirements represent yet another ill-conceived bureaucratic burden for them. Other medical educators are concerned that curriculum is window dressing, some vague, idealistic academic dream. So why did the Residency Review Committee change its rules and expectations? Why did it do so when it did? And why the general curriculum frenzy? Its proponents believe in curriculum as an instrument that can make residency education, and potentially all medical education, more relevant, more dynamic, more effective. Something about their belief has taken root, perhaps because the very nature of the curriculum as a concept has changed.

To begin with, although in introducing a requirement for explicit curriculum development the Residency Review Committee had no illusions that these "concise written documents" would, by themselves, take on some kind of magical power to transform residency teaching, the Committee did have certain pragmatic purposes in mind. The rationale for a written curriculum was, first, that the writing of such a document itself pushes the faculty to be extremely clear about the nature, purpose, and expectations for each and every part of the residency. In effect, creating this kind of "experiential curriculum" forces answers to the question: "Why is each experience in the residency important?"

Second, by making explicit the nature and purpose of every rotation, every experience, faculty and residents can agree ahead of time on what to expect, thereby preventing the frustration and disappointment that occur on both sides when there is a mismatch of faculty and resident expectations. And because the expectations in a written curriculum are explicit, these descriptions can serve as concrete benchmarks for residents as they decide whether rotations have "delivered," and for faculty as they decide whether residents have "measured up."

The Special Requirements for internal medicine residency also explicitly indicate that "residents should be involved in creating and revising the [curriculum] document" (1). The rationale here is that participation in the process of curriculum development helps residents make the transition from the more passive role of students (who do what they are told to do) to the active role of professionals (who do what they tell themselves they should do). Besides, by sharing in the responsibility for designing their own education rather than simply accepting what the program has to offer, residents will only be doing what is already standard practice for graduate students in most other fields. Finally, in contrast with implied or implicit curricula, written curriculum documents can be shared, making it easier for program directors, as they should, to borrow each others' best educational ideas rather than requiring each, working in splendid isolation, to re-invent the wheel.

This new requirement also explicitly equates curriculum with clinical experience—any and all clinical experience: "The focus of the written program description should be the residents' patient-based care experiences" (1). In this, the Residency Review Committee makes clear that it has moved beyond the traditional "learning objectives" definition of curriculum beloved of the classroom educator, and has faced up to the realities of clinical education. Alfred North Whitehead is reputed to have said that "Nothing is as useless as a merely well-informed person." It is therefore the task of clinical education to take learners past being "merely well informed" and on into being full-fledged doctors, with the skills and competencies they need to "put it all together," to perform at a high professional level. The Committee understands very well that clinical education operates in the unpredictable world of real clinical settings, not in the artificial structure of the classroom, and through real, if controlled, clinical experiences—in short, it operates through an experiential curriculum (2,3). (See Chapter 10, What Is a Curriculum?)

These residency Special Requirements also treat both the writing of curriculum and the finished curriculum document itself as living elements of the residency rather than as static formalities. That is, in addition to sharing the creation, faculty are expected to share the written curriculum with residents on a regular basis, particularly at the start of new rotations, and to update it from time to time lest it become dusty and irrelevant.

So far so good. It is easy to see, however, why program directors and faculty might, in all good faith, interpret this new curriculum requirement simply as a request to describe their present programs exactly as they are and leave it at that. This raises the unfortunate possibility that the new requirement might produce nothing more than "snapshots" of the status quo, thus highlighting a key assumption by the Residency Review Committee that curriculum is—and should be—precisely the opposite: a lever for change. Otherwise, why bother with it? An exercise that isn't a powerful and useful instrument for changing residency education will indeed be little more than bureaucratic window dressing.

Stated differently, a curriculum may be said to be most useful when it drives the setting of priorities. Three years of residency experience is a very short time in which to become an independent professional. Unfortunately, residents' roles and experiences are all too often dictated by what teaching sites are most easily available and most familiar to the faculty, not to mention in need of service or "coverage." At the extreme, much of residents' experience may be related to such peripheral or highly specialized services that their thinking takes on a strange and distorted character; for example, as one resident said, half jokingly, "When a patient complains of abdominal pain, rejection of their liver transplant should be number one in your differential." Deciding on priorities—that is, the relative educational value—of the various experiences residents may be exposed to is thus both a crucial and an extremely difficult job, and priority setting is very much what curriculum is all about (4). (See Chapter 13, Content Matters.)

But how will program directors know how to write such a document? They'll need to know what elements should go into it; they'll need to understand what descriptions will provide the most powerful and useful leverage for improvement, if curriculum is to deliver on its many implied promises.

To address these questions, a group of thirteen program directors met over several months in Philadelphia in 1993, to think through for themselves the meaning and uses of curriculum, its elements, and its language. At its first meeting, the group decided it wanted to move quickly to writing. Equally quickly, however, it decided not to begin by describing an existing residency rotation; they were concerned that the administrative, logistic, and psychological freight associated with familiar rotations would make it difficult to define the rationale and expectations they were looking for in a "better" rotation. Accordingly, they took on as their first homework assignment a written response to the following request: "You have just learned you have a vacant month in your schedule and have decided to create a cardiology elective to fill this time. Write a concise curriculum that describes this elective."

Eight of the thirteen program directors did their homework. All of the curricula were concise; all were thoughtful and rich in ideas; many elements were common among them, many were unique. While the final implications of this curriculum "starter set" remain to be worked out, several things are already clear. Many program directors felt it was important for their curriculum to be specific about particular diseases or problem domains that should be mastered, a kind of core clinical problem list (e.g., "know how to diagnose and manage unstable angina, aortic stenosis" and the like), thus forcing choices of specific patients to be cared for, when and if such an elective were actually implemented. Others were specific about responsibilities (e.g., consulting versus primary responsibility for patients), thus forcing choice of clerkship sites and roles. Still others focused on skills to be acquired (e.g., aspects of the cardiovascular physical examination, reading ECGs, performing treadmill tests), thus forcing choices of tasks.

Perhaps most interesting of all, one program director reported that he and his colleagues started out with the homework as a paper exercise, but wound up being so pleased with the curriculum they had created that they actually went ahead and started it. Talk about leverage for change!

At subsequent meetings, discussion of these curriculum proposals eventually led to a consideration of the teaching techniques and elements of the teaching environment that should be included in an "ideal" cardiology elective, since it was clear that description of clinical experience, however detailed, would not answer the question "What makes learning happen?" This discussion opened a new dimension of clinical education beyond the experience of patient care itself. It led to considerations of the pace or timing of teaching, of opportunities to break down complex tasks into parts, of opportunities to synthesize individual skills and knowledge into wholes, of the value of learning by teaching other people, and of the need to couple experience with reflection and concept building. In fact, it opened the possibility that the question of what makes any clinical learning happen—expert learning, in particular—may be the very question for which, ultimately, curriculum is the answer (3). (See Chapter 24, The Right Hand of Claude.)

REFERENCES

1. **Accreditation Council for Graduate Medical Education.** Revised Special Requirements for Residency Training Programs in Internal Medicine. Graduate Medical Education Directory. Chicago: American Medical Association; 1993.
2. **Ende J, Davidoff F.** What is a curriculum? Ann Intern Med. 1992;116:1055-7.
3. **Kolb DA.** Experiential Learning. Experience as the Source of Learning and Development. Englewood Cliffs, NJ: PTR Prentice Hall; 1984.
4. **Davidoff F.** Rethinking graduate medical education: Is a relative educational value scale possible? In: Proceedings of the Second HRSA Primary Care Conference, March 21–23, 1990. Washington, D.C.: U.S. Department of Health and Human Services, Public Health Services, Health Resources and Services Administration; 1990:233-63.

CHAPTER *10*

What Is a Curriculum?

[Jack Ende, MD, and Frank Davidoff, MD]

*T*he Residency Review Committee for Internal Medicine is poised to issue a new requirement that core programs develop a "written curriculum." This event, together with increasing attention to curriculum in the medical literature (1,2) and the recent Association of Professors in Medicine–Association of American Medical Colleges Retreat on the Internal Medicine Residency Curriculum, signals a new direction for medical residencies. Viewing housestaff programs as enterprises for hospital-based service is increasingly unacceptable; these programs must now be conceived of principally in terms of education. And although it is naive to assume that service will diminish in importance for residency training programs, the structure of the programs will clearly have to be recast.

An important step in that recasting will be the development of curricula. There is a sense that internal medicine residency training programs are plagued with problems and that within new curricula will lie at least some of the solutions. We agree with this concept (3) but suggest that before we all rush forward like the character in one of Stephen Leacock's comic novels, who "flung himself upon his horse and rode madly off in all directions," we might consider the more fundamental question, "What is a curriculum?"

Editor's Note: This chapter originally appeared in an education supplement of *Annals of Internal Medicine* (1992;116:1055-7). The question it explores—what is a curriculum?—is even more relevant today, as internal medicine considers the role that can be played by central organizations such as the Federated Council of Internal Medicine, in what ultimately remains a local, deliberative curriculum development process.

WHAT IS A CURRICULUM?

Of the three major branches of education—curriculum, instruction, and evaluation—curriculum is the most difficult to define. Even experts disagree on its basic meaning (4,5). For our purposes, we will start with the definition of curriculum as a plan that will determine an educational experience. Such a definition, however, leaves open as many issues as it closes. What will that plan look like? Will it resemble the highly detailed lesson plan of a classroom teacher, or will it be more like a mission statement used to guide a discussion group? What will be used as the basic building materials of the curriculum? Will it be constructed from lists of behaviors that all learners are to acquire, or will it be assembled from the experiences that all learners are to have? And what purposes will the curriculum serve? Will it be designed to ensure that all learners achieve a level of competence in a certain domain, or will it be intended to serve as a lever to manipulate a societal problem, similar to the way math and science curricula were intended to close the perceived nationwide technology "gap" during the post-Sputnik era?

These questions are not merely theoretical. In the absence of a well-defined concept of what curriculum is and what it is intended to accomplish, we might reasonably ask whether the requirement for a written curriculum will mean anything. What will faculty be expected to write down? How will the curriculum be helpful? Many program directors and department chairs have had experience with curricula generated at great expenditure of faculty effort and time, yet that effort in the end seemed to count for little. How can we ensure that a new curriculum actually will be used and will lead to better trained residents?

THE TRADITIONAL CURRICULUM MODEL

Perhaps something can be learned from those well-crafted curricula that rest peacefully in program directors' bottom desk drawers. Most written curricula for internal medicine residency programs have been fashioned from the traditional or technologic model (5,6) of curriculum. Here the curriculum maker first determines the knowledge and skills the learners are expected to acquire and then determines the knowledge and skills they already possess. The difference between what is and what *is expected* is parceled into discrete learning objectives, those "at the end of the course the learner will be able to do . . ." statements with which we have all become familiar. The objectives determine the mode of instruction and are used further to evaluate the program's success. Curricula formed in this way possess an internal, almost seductive logic. So what, then, is wrong with this approach?

The concern that education theorists would raise, that this approach is excessively teacher-dominated, seems less relevant to our world than a more pressing concern: For graduate medical education, this model simply does not fit. Graduate medical education, by design, takes place in relatively uncontrolled but high-fidelity situations, the real world of clinical care. Graduate education is concerned with complex, multidimensional goals that are difficult to parcel out. How can one describe meaningfully by learning objectives all that is required for "working at the fuzzy boundaries of medical knowledge" (6)—as, for example, in managing a patient with chronic fatigue syndrome—and for achieving the level of diagnostic insight, conscientiousness, humanism, and integrity to which we hope our trainees will aspire? Learning objectives and other reductionistic approaches to curriculum may make sense in well-controlled classroom settings, where core knowledge and skill can be readily identified; but that description hardly applies to programs for housestaff training. Eisner, who is not a physician, reminds us that (7)

> the point here is not to inject the mystical into educational planning but rather to avoid the reductionistic thinking that impoverishes our view of what is possible.

TURNING THE PROBLEM UPSIDE DOWN—THE ESSENTIALS OF GRADUATE MEDICAL EDUCATION

Perhaps we will get a better view if we turn the problem upside down. Rather than impose on graduate medical education a less than appropriate model of curriculum, we should perhaps first examine the realities of residency training and then cast a model of curriculum that will fit. One does not mold clay with scissors or channel a stream with a straightedge. Nor should we try to reorient residency training programs with a model of curriculum that ignores the essentials of that experience, which include important characteristics of the environment, the nature of clinical problem solving, and the process by which residents learn.

Stripped to its essentials, residency training is a series of experiences with patients that occurs in a "real world" learning environment. That environment is no more predictable than the next admission from the emergency room and no more orderly than a night on call. Yet this environment can be enormously educational, even if the lessons that residents learn are not all "in the books." The patient who has crushing chest pain but refuses admission to the cardiac care unit, the patient with hypertension who cannot afford medications—these are the experiences of residency, experiences that Schön (8) would characterize as "configurations of uncertainty, disorder, and indeterminacy." Yet these same experiences become the building blocks of the residency curriculum.

How physicians learn to handle these situations is only recently becoming understood (9–12). Suffice it to say that the process depends on more than finite knowledge or even pattern recognition. Experienced clinicians are able to recognize certain clues and reconfigure problems in such a way that they suddenly make sense. The point here is that this process cannot be learned by memorization, reading, or lectures. This process requires learning of a different sort.

Learning in graduate medical education begins with an experience, a new clinical encounter that throws into question the learner's previous assumptions (13,14). An alternating process of reflection—or mental exploration of the experience—and action follows (15). The learner thinks about the experience, appreciates more about it than he or she did before, takes action, examines the consequences of the action, and so on. The mentor or teacher plays an instrumental role at this stage (16). Experiential learning usually takes place in a social context and depends on the nature of the experience, the skill of the teacher in stimulating reflection, and, of course, the characteristics of the learner for successful assimilation. Previous knowledge is critical—one cannot think about things one does not know—but knowledge in this model of learning is not so much received as discovered. In sum, clinical learning is "experience examined." The experience alone is not clinical education, it is service; the examining alone is not clinical education, it is pedantry.

Given the unpredictable environment of residency training, the nature of the problems residents must learn to solve, and the process that best describes how they learn, understanding why the technologic model of curriculum is less than ideal becomes easy. The problem with the technologic model is that it specifies the outcome but uncouples the outcome from the process, which is where the learning actually occurs. However, in turning away from this particular model of curriculum, we are not turning away from curriculum per se. To say that a set of objectives cannot be specified in advance for a rotation in a residency training program is one thing. To say we should entirely abandon the concept of educational purpose is quite another statement. The question is therefore, "How can that purpose best be described and how can it best be achieved?"

AN EXPERIENTIAL CURRICULUM

We favor an approach to curriculum that formally accepts the experiences that residents will have as basic building blocks. These experiences include interactions with patients, peers, co-workers, and faculty, at the bedside, in the office, and in the conference room. A major advantage of this model of curriculum is that the essentials of residency training—the environment, experiences, and process of learning—are all explicitly included and receive the attention they deserve.

Curriculum development, according to the experiential model, takes place as a deliberative process (17) in which all stakeholders are involved. The stakeholders—faculty, residents, and support staff—must identify, first in general terms and then with increasing degrees of specificity, what they value most in residency training. They must bring their educational values to the table, find common ground, and then choose the types of experiences they believe will truly reflect these values. (Indeed, the term *value choice* might describe this model of curriculum at least as well as *experiential.*) In effect, for each experience, the group must answer the questions "What do we really feel will be the value of residents having this experience?" and "How does that value measure up to the other experiences they could be having?" Simply "placing" residents in available working sites is not enough; placement—apprenticeship, in effect (18)—forces no educational value choices and asserts no educational control. The curriculum makers must consider and make decisions about modes of instruction and supervision. As part of the resident's experience, these modes become elements of the curriculum as do, of course, the patients the residents will care for.

Choices about the patients the residents will care for play a special role in the experiential model of curriculum; after all, the most important lessons are learned with patients. Although these choices are now driven largely by custom and convenience, they could be made on a more rational basis. Thus, as suggested elsewhere (see Chapter 13, Content Matters) (19), methods already exist that should make it possible to articulate the educational values attached to individual pathophysiologic states, diseases, and types of medical encounter through the creation of an explicit, data-based, "relative educational value scale."

At the same time, we cannot simply assume that all of the knowledge residents need will be encompassed by their experiences in caring for patients. Exposure to important, "not-to-be-missed" diagnoses and to more general, cross-cutting subjects can be assured only through organized didactic experiences, where examination of anticipated experience occurs through active participation in workshops, seminars, and the like. Thus, curriculum makers will have to consider the entire range of knowledge and skill that all residents should acquire, either through experience, reading, or discussion. In contrast to the technologic theory of curriculum, in which lists of knowledge and skills represent final destinations, in the experiential model of curriculum the lists provide only points of departure.

Creating residency curricula that are based on the experiential model will be a challenge. The process of explicitly defining and choosing educational values is time-consuming and is not familiar to many faculty and residents. Programmatic changes based on choices made among educational values may threaten entrenched interests such as service needs, departmental status, and so forth. And, to the extent that the curriculum development effort focuses on description of existing experiences rather than on choice among educational values, the model can become an apologia for a less than satisfactory status quo.

The advantages of an experiential curriculum model, however, are many. The model is sufficiently broad to encompass the richness and complexity of residency experience. If we acknowledge that the realities of residency training are as important as the abstractions of knowledge content, it is clear that the experiential model is both pragmatic and unique to each residency site. But although the model is grounded in the realities of residency training, those realities are not regarded as immutable. Rather, use of the model forces those realities into clear focus, enabling them to be molded to the model's purpose. Working back and forth between the curriculum makers' values and the programs' realities allows for educational choices that are explicit and hence documentable, which is useful to faculty, residents, and accrediting bodies alike.

CONCLUSION

We agree that the development of curricula will be an important contribution to the improvement of internal medicine residencies. First, however, we must answer the basic question, "What is the most appropriate curriculum model for clinical training?" An experiential model may serve the purpose, or at the very least, provide a starting point for the discussion and debate that will be necessary to create the model best suited to medical residency training.

REFERENCES

1. **Barker LR.** Curriculum for ambulatory care training in medical residency: rationale, attitudes, and generic proficiencies. J Gen Intern Med. 1990;5(1 Suppl):S3-14.
2. **Association of Program Directors in Internal Medicine.** Careers in Internal Medicine. 1991;7:10.

3. Davidoff F. Medical residencies: quantity or quality? [editorial]. Ann Intern Med. 1989;110:757-8.
4. McNeil JD. Curriculum: A Comprehensive Introduction. Boston: Little, Brown; 1985.
5. Eisner EW, Vallance E. Conflicting Conceptions of Curriculum. Berkeley, CA: McCutchon Publishing Co.; 1974:1-18.
6. Kassirer JP. Clinical problem-solving: a new feature in the Journal. N Engl J Med. 1992;326:60-1.
7. Eisner EW. The Educational Imagination: On the Design and Evaluation of School Programs. 2nd ed. New York: Macmillan; 1985:115.
8. Schön DA. Educating the Reflective Practitioner: Toward a New Design for Teaching and Learning in the Professions. San Francisco: Jossey-Bass; 1988.
9. Perkins DN, Solomon G. Are cognitive skills context-bound? Educational Researcher. January–February 1989:16-25.
10. Schmidt HG, Norman GR, Boshuizen HP. A cognitive perspective on medical expertise: theory and implications. Acad Med. 1990;65:611-21.
11. Elstein AS, Shulman LS, Sprafka SA. Medical Problem Solving: An Analysis of Clinical Reasoning. Cambridge, MA: Harvard University Press; 1978.
12. Bordage G, Lemieux M. Semantic structures and diagnostic thinking of experts and novices. Acad Med. 1991;66(9 Suppl):S70-2.
13. Kolb DA. Experiential Learning. Experience at the Source of Learning and Development. Englewood Cliffs, NJ: Prentice Hall; 1984.
14. Jarvis P. Adult Learning in the Social Context. London: Croom Helm; 1987.
15. Brookfield SD. Understanding and Facilitating Adult Learning. San Francisco: Jossey-Bass; 1990.
16. Daloz L. Effective Teaching and Mentoring. San Francisco: Jossey-Bass; 1986.
17. Atkins E. A sensible faculty-designed model for curriculum development. Journal of Curriculum and Supervision. 1991;6:312-24.
18. Ludmerer KM. Learning to Heal: The Development of American Medical Education. New York: Basic Books; 1985.
19. Davidoff F. Rethinking graduate medical education: Is a relative educational value scale possible? In: Proceedings of the Second HRSA Primary Care Conference, March 21–23, 1990. Washington, D.C.: U.S. Department of Health and Human Services, Public Health Services, Health Resources and Services Administration; 1990:233-63.

CHAPTER *11*

Mirror, Mirror

Medicine Enters the Self-Assessment Era

Mirror, mirror on the wall, who's the fairest one of all?

THE WICKED QUEEN, IN *SNOW WHITE*

*T*he mirror is the prototype of self-assessment instruments. For some decades now, physicians in the United States have been able to look at themselves in self-assessment mirrors, which makes it possible for them to examine the state of their medical knowledge, warts and all, and compare themselves with their peers on a national scale. If professionalism implies continuing self-improvement through self-knowledge (1), then self-assessment is the right thing for medicine to be doing, even though the resulting view may not be flattering.

The launching of the knowledge self-assessment era in medicine first required the development of nondistorting "mirrors for the mind"; they have not always been available. It is easy to forget that as recently as the beginning of this century, most formal medical teaching in the United States consisted of lectures, since the "case history" as a method of teaching had not yet been invented. Walter Cannon, who introduced the case method into medical teaching around the year 1900, commented at the time on an unanticipated and somewhat perplexing feature of this innovation, namely, "that of showing to the students themselves and also to their instructor what they do not know and wherein their knowledge is inaccurate (2)." The case method thus emerged as an early self-assessment instrument, one of the first "mirrors for the mind."

Starting about 1915, medicine in the United States adopted specialty board certification as its new paradigm of professionalism. Certification has continued to grow and flourish to the present day, becoming yet another important reflector of the state of physicians' medical knowledge. What certification delivers to its participants, however, is a summary judgment (a "summative" measurement, to use the educational jargon), a backward look at where your knowledge has gotten to, in contrast to other self-assessment programs that deliver a working reflection (a "formative" measurement), a view toward the future intended primarily as the basis for moving your knowledge forward. In other words, certification tells people whether they measure up but doesn't let them know the criteria against which they were judged. It says, in effect: "Either you know the answers or you don't. The result, if you don't, is that you are assigned to the category of the less knowledgeable."

The certification paradigm flows from the simple reality that creation of a defensible passing standard in a "high-stakes" certifying process requires the use of a secured examination, one that in internal medicine, at least, is made up almost exclusively of multiple-choice questions. Since the content of the examination is confidential, the results obviously can't be used to tell candidates exactly where and why they didn't pass. Thus, board certification itself can't serve to close the educational feedback loop, but rather plays an educational role largely by serving as a motivator and guide to learning captured in the now-familiar admonition, "This might be on the boards."

The first formal, systematic working reflector of medical knowledge was the American College of Physicians' "Medical Knowledge Self-Assessment Program" (MKSAP). MKSAP, which is designed for general internists and covers all of internal medicine and related disciplines, began simply as sets of multiple-choice questions but has evolved into a complex program that, in addition to the questions, now contains syllabus text, annotated bibliographies, and more. Importantly, the program also gives users a specific learning objective plus a written critique of all the answers, right and wrong, and a literature reference for each of the questions. First published in 1968, MKSAP, curiously enough, wasn't conceived of initially as a way of providing direct feedback to its users on the state of their knowledge. In fact, the initial judgment of its designers was that MKSAP scores would be such strong stuff that they wouldn't be useful to individual physicians; more specifically, they were concerned that the College's member internists simply wouldn't be willing to confront their knowledge deficits.

The concept was, rather, that MKSAP scores would be useful to the

College's Education Committee by telling them what internists don't know, thus providing guidance on which continuing education programs were needed (3). As the program evolved, however, faith in the ability of the College's membership to handle information about knowledge deficits grew to the point where it was decided not only to give users their own scores, but also to tell them exactly which questions they got wrong. Ironically, MKSAP was later almost killed because of concern that members' low scores could be extremely damaging if they fell into the hands of patients, colleagues, and others. The program was eventually allowed to proceed but only after it was hedged around with extensive safeguards to protect the confidentiality of individual performance scores.

Despite all the concern about its power, the essence of self-assessment is extraordinarily simple; it is the notion that learning by asking yourself a question is fundamentally different from, and more meaningful than, learning by memorizing a fact. Thus, while the initial concerns of the MKSAP developers focused around the judgments implicit in all test scores, the true power of self-assessment lies not in the scores themselves but in how people respond to the information they receive on their answers to individual questions. Such detailed, specific feedback allows participants to judge for themselves, on the basis of their own standards, the state of their own medical knowledge and, based on that feedback, to do something specific about it. Thus, in contrast with the summative judgments produced by certification, the self-assessment paradigm says: "Either you know the answer or you don't. Finding out exactly what you don't know puts you in a strong position to learn it." While not expressed in quite the same terms as the rallying cry of Continuous Quality Improvement, "Every defect is a treasure," the self-assessment paradigm has, in effect, been saying exactly that for a long time.

One internist's experience in Albania highlights the unique strengths of self-assessment as a model of the kind of critical questioning that is so much taken for granted in U.S. medical education, including, increasingly, in continuous lifelong learning (W.G.M. Hardison, personal communication). (See Chapter 7, Lifelong Learning.) Medical education in many parts of the world is authoritarian, but in Albania during the Soviet era it had become absolutely and rigidly autocratic; what professors taught was truth. So when Hardison arrived to spend the year 1994–95 as visiting faculty in Tirana, he quickly found that his best efforts to persuade Albanian medical students and residents to question medical evidence were met with little more than bewilderment. As time went by, however, he noticed that his students and residents were particularly attracted to the self-assessment programs he had brought with him, and used them increasingly; they were then able to move progressively from self-questioning to raising questions more generally. For these learners, self-assessment effectively modeled the deceptively simple concept of learning by questioning, serving as a bridge from passive acceptance to active critical inquiry.

The evidence that medicine has entered the self-assessment era is all around us.

- First, it's pervasive. Most medical specialty societies now provide their members with self-assessment programs.

- Second, residents are using it. Residents in most medical disciplines participate in some form of in-training examination. While on the surface these exercises look like tests (largely multiple-choice questions), most are designed to be used, and in internal medicine, are used, in a formative, educational, self-assessment mode, rather than in a summative, categorizing mode.

- Third, it has established a place within recertification. Recertification in internal medicine includes a major self-assessment component, the Self-Evaluation Process, or SEP (4). While the American Board of Internal Medicine is careful to point out that the SEP will not, by itself, be an educational exercise, the Board generally views recertification as important in fostering a key component of clinical competence –that is, continuing scholarship. Thus, for the first time, the summative certification paradigm in internal medicine will be directly paired within the same program with the formative, educational self-assessment paradigm.

- Fourth, the Residency Review Committee in Internal Medicine now recommends it. As of 1994, the Special Requirements for Residency Training Programs in Internal Medicine explicitly support the use of self-assessment instruments and exercises.

- Fifth, the subspecialty societies in internal medicine, many of which had over the years developed their own self-assessment instruments, are collaborating with the American College of Physicians to produce a series of ten Subspecialty MKSAPs, each devoted exclusively to a subspecialty area.

Self-assessment of medical knowledge has thus become an enduring element of medical professionalism, a major expression of the principle that "The one unchanging feature of the professional is unceasing movement toward new levels of performance (1)." And while the principal standard by which that professionalism is judged is still the profession's own definition of what level of medical knowledge is acceptable, the patient's definition of an acceptable level of medical practice is also being recognized as an appropriate and relevant standard (5). Indeed, nondistorting "mirrors" that reflect patients' perceptions of the nature and level of care back to physicians, nurses, administrators, and others are actively being developed and used (6). The self-assessment era in medicine, in this broader sense, may be just beginning.

REFERENCES

1. **Nowlen PM.** A New Approach to Continuing Education in Business and the Professions. New York: Collier Macmillan; 1988:11.
2. **Reiser SJ.** The clinical record in medicine. Part 1: Learning from cases. Ann Intern Med. 1991;114:902-7.
3. **Davidoff F.** The American College of Physicians and the Medical Knowledge Self-Assessment paradigm. Journal of Continuing Education in Health Professions. 1989;9:233-8.
4. **Glassock RJ, Benson JA Jr, Copeland RB, Godwin HA Jr, Johanson WG Jr, Point W, et al.** Time-limited certification and recertification: the program of the American Board of Internal Medicine. The Task Force on Recertification. Ann Intern Med. 1991;114:59-62.
5. **Moloney TW, Paul B.** The consumer movement takes hold in medical care. Health Aff (Millwood). 1991;10:268-79.
6. **Cleary PD, Edgman-Levitan S, Roberts M, Moloney TW, McMullen W, Walker JD, et al.** Patients evaluate their hospital care: a national survey. Health Aff (Millwood). 1991;10:254-67.

PART Two

FEELINGS

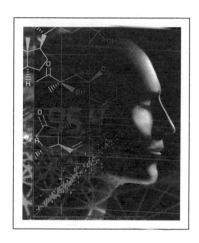

CHAPTER 12

The Dilemma
of the Uninteresting Patient

*H*ere's the dilemma:

- All doctors would rather deal with interesting rather than uninteresting medical problems.
- Many patients' problems, particularly in general internal medicine practice, are seen as uninteresting.
- How can doctors learn, as they must, to make the uninteresting interesting?

A generalist is essentially defined by the expectation that he or she will take an interest in whatever a patient brings through the door; in a word, by the inclusiveness of his or her practice. Specialists and subspecialists, in contrast, have the luxury of declaring they're not interested in one or another of the patient's problems, and sending the patient off somewhere else—most likely to a generalist. In fact, a medical specialty is defined precisely by the exclusivity of its interests, drawing much of its strength from this very ability to exclude attention to most problems so it can concentrate on a few.

Finding all patients (and their problems) interesting is also the basis for continued relationships with patients over time, another hallmark of generalist practice. Writing over twenty years ago, the British psychiatrist Michael Balint eloquently captured this crucial aspect of generalism in his comparison of the generalist practitioner with the specialist (in this case, a psychiatrist) (1):

> The latter has only one kind of relationship with his patient. True, it is a rich and highly involved relationship, but it is of one kind. If it is discontinued . . . what can be described . . . as the single thread between them is broken. There is a finality about it that is lacking in the case of the patient of a general practitioner. The relationship between the latter and his patient has numerous threads, and the truer the general practitioner is to his vocation, the stronger and more numerous they are. So the practitioner can take considered risks with his patients, risks which cannot be taken by a psychiatrist. Even if the openly psychotherapeutic relationship [with a general practitioner] is broken off, the patient may, and indeed does, come back to his doctor with a cold, or indigestion, or a whitlow, or a bruised finger, or to have his child inoculated, and so on ad infinitum.

The dilemma is a serious one, and it particularly confronts both practicing general internists and teachers of generalist skills. The challenge presented by this dilemma isn't made any easier by its association with two additional, widely held but misguided assumptions: 1) that certain characteristics of patients and their problems are intrinsically more interesting than others; and 2) that physicians' interest in patients' problems derives largely from the physician's own personality and previous experience, implying that interest isn't teachable.

Now, it's not hard to figure out what characteristics make patients seem intrinsically "interesting." Think about comments heard every day in the hospital corridor, such as: "I saw the most interesting patient recently . . . ." In such cases, it's a pretty safe bet that the speaker is referring to a patient with a problem that is rare, atypical, or exotic; unexplained or mysterious; moderately complex rather than very simple or hopelessly tangled; acute rather than chronic; severe rather than mild; and curable.

Fascination with such characteristics is not, of course, confined to medicine. At the very least, the fascination probably has something to do with preventing boredom. It may also reflect something even deeper—the very ability to stay in touch with reality. As Robert Pirsig, author of *Zen and the Art of Motorcycle Maintenance*, explains (2, p 247):

> *Any* intellectually conceived object is *always* in the past and therefore *unreal*. Reality is always the moment of vision *before* the intellectualization takes place. *There is no other reality.*

Newness, change, variety, rarity, freshness, mystery—all bring us closer to this special awareness of the "moment of vision," to what Pirsig has called Quality. And internal medicine, that most intellectual of disciplines, may be particularly vulnerable to losing contact with Quality (2, p 247):

> [I]ntellectuals usually have the greatest trouble seeing this Quality, precisely because they are so swift and absolute about snapping everything into intellectual form.

The patient that is interesting to our hospital corridor commentator is also likely to be younger rather than older; physically attractive rather than deformed, old, or ugly; compliant rather than demanding or careless; stoical rather than complaining. In this complex "interest-defining equation," therefore, the patient as a person figures at least as heavily as the patient's problem.

The assumption that people in general, and physicians in particular, can't or won't learn to make uninteresting things interesting is understandable. However, a variety of skills and attitudes such as empathy that were traditionally seen as nonteachable or unlearnable have already yielded to new conceptual models and teaching approaches (3). It would seem prudent, therefore, to reserve judgment on the question of whether physicians can learn to make patients interesting, and whether patients are born or made interesting.

Our understanding of what makes patients interesting is obviously still primitive. However, even at this early stage of understanding, a few rather pragmatic operating principles can be identified as the basis for teaching in this vexing but crucial area (4).

1. **Interest is in the mind of the beholder.** One physician's yawn is another's fascinoma. While, as noted above, certain kinds of patients and their problems are more likely to be seen as interesting, it is clear that the quality of interesting-ness resides in physicians' minds. Although physicians have little control over their patients' characteristics, they can, in theory at least, influence what goes on inside their own heads. It does not seem unrealistic, therefore, to conclude that the skill of making patients interesting is teachable and learnable. The obligation to find your patients interesting is also arguably part of medical professionalism; acquiring the skill of making patients interesting should thus be an absolute requirement of medical education. (See Chapter 28, Heart and Head.)

2. **All patients are interesting.** This statement would be a prime candidate for a "Generalists' Creed." Just as it is arguably true that "the

only normal patient is the patient who has not been tested," it is even more likely to be true that "the only uninteresting patient is the one nobody has tried to make interesting." But lest this "Creed" be taken as self-righteous or preachy, it may be useful to add (in parentheses), "But some patients are a little more interesting than others." (See Chapter 29, A Technology for Remembering.)

3. **All patients are interesting to themselves.** A patient who has lost all interest in himself or herself is probably either suicidally depressed or comatose. Loss of interest in yourself may be closely related to the serious problem of loss of identity, as Erik Erikson pointed out many years ago. Thus, while a physician can't be expected to have the same interest in a patient as the patient himself or herself, patients are exquisitely sensitive to physicians' apparent lack of interest in them. A patient's statement that "My doctor didn't seem interested in me" is a warning of serious impending trouble.

4. **All patients are interesting as people.** It is one thing to see twenty different cases of diabetes in the course of a week; it is quite another to see twenty different people as patients, all of whom happen to have diabetes. In every case, the very same biological disease "lives" in a different person, and the disease expresses itself differently in every one of them. Learning about what makes these individual patients "tick," biologically and psychologically; figuring out how best to interact with each of them; deciding how best to negotiate, to develop therapeutic alliances, to use language effectively—all provide potentially endless sources of interest. Even patients who are "difficult"—demanding, disorganized, hateful—can be approached using a variety of important interest-generating techniques, particularly the approach known as "mining for gold," that is, searching around until you find some redeeming feature as a starting point for a working relationship (5).

5. **Think like patients.** This admonition has nothing whatsoever to do with recreating the patient's thoughts in your mind. Rather, the task thus described is "putting your mind inside the patient's situation," in effect eliminating the gap between you as a health care worker and the medical work you are trying to do. Describing someone who is working in this mode, Pirsig writes (2, p 296):

One says of him that he is "interested" in what he's doing, that he's "involved" in his work. What produces this involvement is, at the cutting edge of consciousness, an absence of any sense of separateness of subject and object.

Lest this formulation be seen as a bit too New Age, it may help to know that it precisely echoes the perspective of Barbara McClintock, who won the Nobel Prize for her work in the genetics of corn. Asked how she achieved such a deep understanding of the subject her comment was: "You have to learn to think like corn." Looked at this way, even a problem as uninteresting on the surface as urinary incontinence in the elderly can blossom into a lifelong interest, once you begin to "think like incontinence," and come to discover its intricate pathophysiology, its enormous psychological, social, and economic impact, and the true sophistication demanded of physicians for high-quality diagnostic workup and therapy of the problem (6).

Dilemmas are frustrating, but meditating on them, like the *koans* of Zen, can and does produce unexpected, useful—and interesting—results.

REFERENCES

1. **Balint M.** The Doctor, His Patient and the Illness. New York: International Universities Press; 1972:158.
2. **Pirsig RM.** Zen and the Art of Motorcycle Maintenance. New York: William Morrow and Co.; 1974.
3. **Platt FW, Keller VF.** Empathic communication: a teachable and learnable skill. J Gen Intern Med. 1994;9:222-6.
4. **Davidoff F.** Five dilemmas in general medicine. SREPCIM Newsletter. 1984;6:1-8.
5. **Levinson W.** Mining for gold. J Gen Intern Med. 1993;8(3):172.
6. **Beck JC, ed.** Geriatrics Review Syllabus: A Core Curriculum in Geriatric Medicine. New York: American Geriatrics Society; 1991: 75-90.

CHAPTER 13

Content Matters

~~~

A Relative Educational Value Scale Considered

*F*or decades, reformers have deplored medical education's preoccupation with content. Thus, the crusading 1984 Report on the General Professional Education of the Physician (GPEP) begins with the flat-footed statement that "the student and the teacher, not the curriculum, are the crucial elements in the educational program," and its first recommendation bemoans the excessive preoccupation with "knowledge" (1). Medical information changes so rapidly that it is appropriate to be wary of excessive concentration on today's received medical wisdom. And no one would disagree that medical education needs to concentrate less on memorization of facts—content acquisition in its most primitive aspect—and, in the process, get better at helping students acquire the complex mental models they'll need for high-level problem solving.

But, at the same time, content-averse logic like this is troubling. Skilled professionals of every kind—lawyers, architects, agronomists, auto mechanics—learn to solve complex, subtle, sophisticated problems, but that doesn't mean they should all be practicing medicine. However difficult the idea may be for educational reformers to accept, physicians are distinguished from other professionals precisely by their knowledge, that is, the specific *content* of the problems they can solve, rather than by any special or unique problem-solving ability; in a word, by *what* they know (and know how to do), not *how* they come to know (and know how to do).

Given the importance of curriculum, it is curious that medical curriculum content, both in medical schools and residencies, has been
determined by social and political forces in the academic marketplace as
much as by any rational, data-driven process. National influences are at
work here: medical school and residency program accreditation standards, certifying board examinations, and information sharing among
faculty, both publicly at national meetings, and, less visibly, through
person-to-person contacts. But, of course, medical education happens
locally; local forces, including precedent and historical accident, local
law and culture, faculty expertise and interests, and locally available
resources, such as training sites and patients, are key determinants of
what residents and students actually experience, and hence the content
of what they learn. Despite its many nationally shared characteristics,
therefore, all medical curriculum is local, in the same sense that all politics is local.

(Remarkably enough, medical school faculty have not until recently
been able to say exactly *what* their students were actually exposed to in
the curriculum, since each class, course, rotation, or experience was
designed by a separate person, group, committee, or department. No
one person or office had a handle on all of the curriculum's component
parts at once, so no one was in a position to add it all up. Computer
tracking systems have now made it possible to collect and synthesize
information about [nearly] everything that is taught; it is at last beginning to be possible to say what content actually is in a medical school's
curriculum.)

Buffeted by these crosscurrents, medical faculty have tended to fall
back on two principles when it comes to choosing curriculum content:

1. **Teach everything.** Squeeze as much as possible into every hour of
    the learner's time. After all, the argument goes, "If we don't teach it
    now, when will they learn it?"

2. **Free-for-all.** Let every person and department push for what they
    can get. Those who command more respect, more clout, more
    resources generally wind up with more input regarding the choice
    of curriculum content. Or, stated differently, some faculty are more
    successful than others in competing for the principal educational
    currency in the academic marketplace, that is, student and resident
    time. (Can it be entirely accidental that we speak of medical trainees
    "spending" their time in various courses and rotations?)

Why isn't medical curriculum content selected more rationally? As suggested above, part of the explanation is undoubtedly political. But cognitive factors may also be important. For it is generally true that the fundamental task in all information processing is separating signal from noise. Much of research consists of exactly this: deciding what is *not* of interest or importance; and medical editors spend much of their time deciding what to *leave out* of journals and books. And since there is a great deal of noise (i.e., an enormous wealth of information available) in the medical education environment, the task of developing curriculum—deciding what is signal and what is noise—is a difficult one when looked at purely from the information-processing point of view.

The emotional side of the problem is at least as important, since deciding to leave things out becomes a matter of setting priorities, which immediately touches on values and on self-esteem. In the specific case of choosing curriculum content, decisions move quickly from *what* topics are more important, to *whose* topics are more important. The need to set priorities translates into accepting the hard reality that some things are more worth learning than others. The logic here is straightforward enough, but the emotional price of priority setting is significant: understandably, everyone thinks of their chosen field as signal; it is painful to think of it as noise.

Now, as faculty we have been highly successful at setting concrete, specific curriculum priorities *within* individual clinical fields: deciding what is important to teach about the tying of surgical knots, for example, or the administration of digitalis, or manipulation of angioplasty catheters. Likewise, we are good at teaching what does and does not matter *within* research: how to choose a research question, design an experiment, collect and interpret data. But despite these successes, we have somehow not yet been able to come up with robust, sophisticated methodologies for setting priorities across an entire curriculum, for deciding which specific clinical problems and what research topics are worth teaching at all.

This problem can't be unique to medicine. Somewhere there must be lessons to be learned about rational ways to assign priorities to things whose value has historically "floated" in a marketplace. An example that immediately comes to mind in this connection is the resource-based relative value scale (RBRVS), which was designed to be an objective and systematic way of assigning values to physician services. Despite the obvious differences between physician services and curriculum content (and ignoring the melancholy political fate of the RBRVS as a method of determining physician reimbursement), we can still find much to learn from the way the RBRVS went about its task (2,3).

In creating its methodology, the RBRVS authors first disaggregated physician services into component parts—that is, the various constituent resources used by physicians in the course of doing their work. These resources included time spent, mental effort and judgment, technical skill, physical effort, and psychological stress; practice costs; and the opportunity costs of specialty training. Second, using physician consensus groups, they quantitated or "weighted" every component of each physician service *within* a specialty using a psychological measurement technique called "magnitude estimation." Third, for each service, they aggregated the weightings assigned to the individual components of each service into an overall score that reflected resource use. Fourth, they chose a "benchmark" service within each specialty, then ranked the overall scores for all services within that specialty relative to the benchmark, thus creating a relative value scale for the entire range of that specialty's services. And, finally, they linked these within-specialty relative value scales across disciplines, using as an anchor the benchmark service from each discipline judged to be equivalent in value to its counterpart benchmark in each of the other disciplines. The final product was a weighted, rank-ordered master list of "resource-based relative values" for all of medical practice.

How could we use this approach to create a medical curriculum? To begin with, and most importantly, we could look at each major disease and health problem in terms of its salient component parts, that is, the features that produce the greatest impact on the greatest number of people: disease or problem frequency; burden of morbidity and mortality; biological and conceptual complexity; difficulty of procedures used in management; degree of physician involvement in usual management; effectiveness of treatment; and resource use (cost). With this information, it should then be possible to create a "relative educational value scale" by using a process analogous to that used in creating the RBRVS (4).

The product would be a list of diseases and health problems. In contrast to most other curriculum documents, however, this would be a *prioritized* list, one which could serve as a rational basis for proportioning out precious curriculum time. The diseases and problems highest on the list would, in effect, become the required or "core" curriculum; those that were lower down would not be lost or dropped, but would become, in effect, electives.

Could this actually be done? A priori the task seems endless, almost intractable. But some medical schools and residencies in this country have already begun to take a broad, integrated look at their curricula in ways that set priorities at least implicitly, if not explicitly and quantitatively. The Medical Council of Canada has generated a list of clinical problems for each major area of medicine that a graduating medical student should be competent to handle; what is not on the list is, by inference, less important (5). And, interestingly, problem-based learning itself—the curriculum reform most closely associated with the learning process, the one generally seen as most stringently divorced from considerations of content—turns out to have developed a set of seven criteria, very similar to those proposed above, for selecting the content (clinical topics) for a problem-based curriculum (6). In fact, problem-based learning has seriously "bitten the curriculum content selection bullet," so much so that skeptics might be forgiven if they concluded that the widespread success of problem-based learning has depended more on improved selection of curriculum content than on the use of new and better learning methods.

Thus, a relative educational value scale might be possible after all. But would it be overkill, not really worth all that faculty time and effort? Can't we set educational priorities through a less fine-grained, exhaustive process? Maybe so. But a "relative educational value scale" could at the very least rationalize medical curriculum to the extent of making content decisions explicit, and hence shared and amenable to critical examination, rather than implicit, as they so often are now. In analogous fashion, the technique of decision analysis now helps rationalize clinical decisions by providing an explicit imaging technique for visualizing them (7). A relative educational value scale would therefore be progress—limited progress perhaps but progress nevertheless, since there is little hope that rational medical curriculum decisions will happen through a process that is primarily socially and politically driven.

REFERENCES

1. **Association of American Medical Colleges.** Project Panel on the General Professional Education of the Physician and College Preparation for Medicine. Physicians for the Twenty-first Century: Report of the Project Panel on the General Professional Education of the Physician and College Preparation for Medicine. Washington, D.C.: Association of American Medical Colleges; 1984.

2. Hsiao WC, Braun P, Yntema D, Becker ER. Estimating physicians' work for a resource-based relative-value scale. N Engl J Med. 1988;319:835-41.
3. Braun P, Yntema DB, Dunn D, DeNicola M, Ketcham T, Verrilli D, Hsiao WC. Cross-specialty linkage of resource-based relative value scales. Linking specialties by services and procedures of equal work. JAMA. 1988;260:2390-6.
4. Davidoff F. Rethinking graduate medical education: Is a relative educational value scale possible? In: Proceedings of the Second HRSA Primary Care Conference, March 21–23, 1990. Washington, D.C.: U.S. Department of Health and Human Services, Public Health Services, Health Resources and Services Administration; 1990:233-63.
5. Bordage G, Page G. An alternative approach to PMPs: the "key features" concept. In: Hart I, Harden R, eds. Further Developments in Assessing Clinical Competence. Proceedings of the Ottawa Conference on Continuing Medical Education. Montreal: Can-Heal Publications; 1987:59-75.
6. Barrows HS, Tamblyn RM. Problem-Based Learning: an Approach to Medical Education. New York: Springer-Verlag; 1980.
7. Davidoff F. Decision analysis: an imaging technique for visualizing medical decisions. In: Nobel J, ed. Textbook of General Medicine and Primary Care. Boston: Little, Brown; 1988:27-34.

CHAPTER 14

Medical Interviewing

The Crucial Skill That Gets Short Shrift

*I*n the course of forty years in practice, an internist can easily expect to participate in at least 200,000 medical interviews, particularly if you include telephone consultations, discussions with patients' families, and the like. This startling figure immediately suggests that several things must be true. First, interviewing must be important. Second, if (as the old joke would have it) the key to doing something well is "practice, practice, practice!", internists must be exceedingly good at it. And third, if we weren't good at it, our patients would have told us so, since they have so many opportunities to do so.

Now, it's hard to deny the importance of medical interviews; they are at the very heart of medicine. By all accounts, the medical interview is the source of at least 80 percent of the specific information needed to arrive at a correct diagnosis in most patients (1). The medical interview also helps physicians build rapport and respond to patients' emotional concerns and is central to education, negotiation, and motivation (2). At the same time, unfortunately, when it comes to medical interviewing even many years of practice don't necessarily make perfect. And, in fact, our patients are making it increasingly clear that there's much room for improvement in how most of us interview (3).

Medical interviewing is one of those paradoxes in life where something seems as though it ought to be simple but turns out not to be. Take running, for example: Nearly everyone can run, so why isn't everyone a professional-level runner? Or, since every doctor can talk and listen, why isn't every one of us skilled at medical interviewing?

Of course, biological and personal differences among physicians account for much of the variation, but the difficulty lies equally with the vast complexity of the interview process itself. In interviewing, as in the arts, what appears to be most artless is, in truth, the result of careful and concentrated effort. Even the seemingly basic elements of medical interviewing are highly sophisticated, and hence difficult for nearly everyone to master. Some of them are

- Getting at the patient's real chief complaint(s)
- Being able to enter the patient's world and perspective without losing sight of the medical issues
- Using language appropriately and well
- "Splitting consciousness" in order to monitor how the interview is going while at the same time remaining connected with the patient

Beyond the basic level, the complexity of medical interviewing is nearly infinite, given the complexity of human beings, their cultures, and their biomedical problems, all of which converge in doctor–patient encounters. The result is that learning high-level medical interviewing skills is both qualitatively and quantitatively different from learning many of the simpler procedural skills. The achievable skill level for most such procedures has a ceiling; that is, you can only get so good at doing them. But it seems there is no real upper limit to excellence in medical interviewing.

At its most difficult, medical interviewing presents many serious challenges: giving bad news, obtaining informed consent, detecting and managing domestic violence, dealing with substance abuse, talking and working with dying patients and their families, managing difficult patients, negotiating advance directives—the list is almost endless. In fact, advanced skill in medical interviewing seems to be the hallmark of "doctors' doctors," most of whom have been, first and foremost, spectacular—even legendary—interviewers of patients.

A particularly challenging aspect of medical interviewing is, of course, that the principal "instrument" of the interview is *ourselves* with all our attendant capabilities of language, mind, and personality, but without the cool objectivity and standardization of the pill, the blade, and the imaging device. Because physicians and patients can't be separated from the interview process itself, the satisfactions, and the frustrations, for both parties are therefore uniquely dependent on a specific set of physician skills. Is it any wonder, then, that it is not easy for everyone to reach and maintain the highest levels of interviewing skill? The curious thing is that anyone at all could think that mastering medical interviewing is as easy as, or easier than, learning most other aspects of medicine.

As with running and other complex professional skills, medical interviewing is better taught and learned through coaching than through conventional methods. The skills of medical interviewing are therefore best learned under "practicum" conditions, rather than in classrooms (4). That practicum needs to include formative feedback such as that from videotaped interviews, interaction with standardized patients, and group observation and discussion, rather than from summative written examinations. And the preferred teacher is a mentor, rather than a lecturer or an attending physician.

Surgeons have long known that the complex realities of operating room surgery can be learned only through practicum experience, in the operating room itself. Long ago, therefore, surgeons in training came to accept the necessity of extensive time in the OR, where every aspect of surgery, from the minutest technical details to the rigorous codes of OR teamwork and etiquette, is enacted and re-enacted in a tight mentoring relationship.

The obvious question is: If medical interviewing matters as much to internists and other generalist physicians as operating room skill does to surgeons, then why don't internists and others in training spend several hours a day with their mentors in the "IR" (i.e., the Interviewing Room), seeing, doing, and teaching interviewing, the way surgeons do with surgery?

Other more general questions quickly follow:

- If medical interviewing is so crucial, why are so little time and emphasis given to it in medical school and residency, particularly relative to other disciplines that may have a great deal less to do with the quality of clinical practice than interviewing does?
- If medical interviewing is so central to the entire enterprise of medical practice, why don't all medical schools have departments of medical interviewing?
- Where is the world-class support you would expect for research in something as important as medical interviewing?
- Why don't a significant number of medical students choose the "specialty" of medical interviewing as the intellectual and academic focus of their careers?
- Why is medical interviewing known in continuing medical education circles as something that "doesn't appeal," and hence is generally avoided?

The simple lack of rationality here is more than a little discouraging, but fortunately for the medical interview and medicine generally, things are looking up a bit. The amount of high-quality research on interviewing is increasing (5,6). A growing number of excellent clinical and scholarly publications, including chapters and textbooks, is available on medical interviewing and related subjects (2,7–9). Many medical schools and residencies are taking a new look at the challenge of teaching and learning medical interviewing (10). And organizations such as the American Academy on Physician and Patient and the Northwest Center for Doctor–Patient Relations devoted exclusively to research, practice, and teaching in medical interviewing have come into being.

The discipline of medical interviewing is far from reaching "critical mass," but these are brave beginnings. Now all that remains is for the rest of the world to take medical interviewing as seriously as it deserves.

REFERENCES

1. **Peterson MC, Holbrook JH, Von Hales D, Smith NL, Staker LV.** Contributions of the history, physical examination, and laboratory investigation in making medical diagnoses. West J Med. 1992;156:163-5.
2. **Cohen-Cole SA.** The Medical Interview: The Three-Function Approach. St Louis: Mosby–Year Book; 1991.
3. **Gerteis M, Edgman-Levitan S, Daley J, Delbanco T, editors.** Through the Patient's Eyes: Understanding and Promoting Patient-Centered Care. San Francisco: Jossey-Bass; 1993.
4. **Schön D.** Educating the Reflective Practitioner: Toward a New Design for Teaching and Learning in the Professions. San Francisco: Jossey-Bass; 1988.
5. **Cassell EJ.** Talking With Patients. Vol. 1: The Theory of Doctor–Patient Communication. Vol. 2: Clinical Technique. Cambridge: MIT Press; 1985.
6. **Roter DL, Hall JA.** Doctors Talking with Patients/Patients Talking with Doctors: Improving Communication in Medical Visits. Westport, CT: Auburn House; 1992.
7. **Billings JA, Stoeckle JD.** The Clinical Encounter: A Guide to the Medical Interview and Case Presentation. Chicago: Year Book Medical Publishers; 1989.
8. **Waitzkin H.** The Politics of Medical Encounters: How Patients and Doctors Deal with Social Problems. New Haven, CT: Yale University Press; 1992.

9. **Lipkin M, Putnam SM, Lazare A, eds.** The Medical Interview: Clinical Care, Education, and Research. New York: Springer-Verlag; 1995.

10. **Novak DH, Volk G, Drossman DA, Lipkin M Jr.** Medical interviewing and interpersonal skills teaching in US medical schools. Progress, problems, and promise. JAMA. 1993;269:2101-5.

CHAPTER 15

Ideals and Motivations

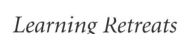

Learning Retreats

L ive, lecture-format continuing medical education (CME) allows people to retreat, if only a little, from the pressures of daily practice, although this isn't CME's principal purpose. In contrast, true learning retreats—not to be confused with traditional CME offered in exotic, "fly-away" packages—are usually held in quiet, secluded locations, involve small groups of learners who essentially teach themselves, with the help of resource people or facilitators, and are specifically intended to be an opportunity to pull away from the pressures of daily work. People who have participated in medical learning retreats often seem to come away with the feeling they have experienced CME at its most "ideal." What is there about learning retreats that touches them so deeply? Is there, in fact, such a thing as "ideal" CME?

The ultimate measure of CME's success is improved patient outcomes, achieved through CME-related changes in clinical practice. But you don't have to be a rocket scientist (as the current saying goes) to figure out that even CME programs offering the most spectacular content in the most effective possible way are unlikely to succeed unless participants are *motivated* to learn and to change their clinical practices. It follows, then, that a great deal more is required of "ideal" CME than that participants are simply provided with passive learning opportunities. It could be that learning retreats seem to people like an ideal way to learn precisely because they are better than other forms of CME at motivating people to learn and change.

Human motivation is complex and mysterious. But one school of thought argues convincingly that three things in particular motivate learning and behavior change: supporting and encouraging *autonomy* (self-initiation), assuring *mastery* (competence), and developing *relatedness* (connection) to other people. Not surprisingly, changes in behavior are not only more likely to happen but are also more likely to be sustained if an education program catalyzes changes by supporting people's need to be self-determining; in contrast, changes brought about by external controls fade when the controls are withdrawn (1).

The social scientist Kurt Lewin is reputed to have said that "There is nothing so practical as a good theory." *Self-determination theory* is a construct developed to describe the relationships among the three elements of learning motivation (2). From the perspective of self-determination theory, learning retreats ought to do a particularly good job of motivating people to learn. But exactly how does this work?

First, retreats by their very nature seem designed to support autonomy and people's "growth-oriented self." The people who come to retreats are, of course, not a random sample, but a self-selected group that is drawn to this kind of "open" learning in the first place. But the basic features of a retreat—isolated location, informal style of living and working, and a duration long enough for participants to come to know each other and to become thoroughly immersed in the content and the process of the retreat—go well beyond the fact of self-selection in this regard. That is, these features all conspire to separate learners from the pressure to do things for other people—patients, colleagues, institutions. Retreats thus support learners' commitment to do something for themselves—not for their personal selves, as during vacations, but for their professional, autonomous, "growth-oriented" selves. Retreats are basically designed to give something to people rather than demand something from them.

Second, good learning retreats make full use of selected learning materials. Articles, chapters, and books are sent out or assigned ahead of time so that the grunt work of getting familiar with the material is done outside the retreat itself. Thus, even before the participants assemble and the retreat actually begins, learners have the opportunity to find out where they're comfortable and where they're stuck—in effect, the participants have gone through a needs assessment like that expected for all good learning. In this instance, however, it's a self-driven needs assessment, which further supports the learners' sense that they're doing this on their own initiative. (See Chapter 34, Continuing Medical Education.)

This pre-retreat exercise does two other useful things: it increases the likelihood that precious time in the retreat will be used for learning, rather than for finding out what people need to learn; and it brings participants together on common intellectual ground right from the start. The retreat itself then consists of working through these assigned materials: sharing insights, exploring confusions, delving deeper into meanings and mechanisms, making sense of issues that didn't make sense before, often learning from the struggles and the insights of other learners. (See Chapter 21, Bankers and Midwives.)

The methods of a retreat thus provide a uniquely potent opportunity for mastering the materials: the give-and-take with colleagues who are working just as hard as you are provides the social stimulus for learning and the intellectual yardstick for testing the limits of your learning—with help from the expert facilitator or resource person as needed. Moreover, the informality and group support in learning retreats can make it safe "not to know," creating an environment where the only "dumb" question is an unasked question—and such an environment is perhaps the single most important condition leading to mastery.

Third, the learners at retreats work closely with each other. Interactive learning in small groups is the exception in most other CME programs. Even in seminar-type CME, the learners tend to interact directly with faculty experts more than with each other. In contrast, much of the group work in good retreats is structured around facilitators whose job is to keep the group together and moving ahead, and from getting too far off the track, but otherwise to stay in the background as much as possible.

Shared professional activity of any kind—reading the same journal as your colleagues or even attending the same lectures—connects people with their profession, albeit the connection is generally with abstract things—for example, the profession's body of knowledge, its culture and values, its codes and practices and traditions. The give-and-take at learning retreats, on the other hand, is concrete and direct, connecting people with the profession as a living, working body of colleagues.

In the context of self-determination theory, then, it is clear why learning retreats might be ideal as a way to motivate learning and change. But this thought brings to mind the old expression "If you're so smart, why aren't you rich?", which translates here into "if learning retreats are so ideal, why aren't they more common?" Perhaps there are hidden problems—trouble in paradise.

In putting together retreats, there is, of course, the need to identify people with both an interest and some experience in organizing CME in this special way, and those people are not always easy to find. Good facilitators aren't always easy to come by, either, and other aspects of learning retreats are problematic as well.

For one thing, ways in which physicians are socialized during their medical school training seem to reinforce their autonomy needs almost to the point of isolation. One group that has carefully studied the process of graduate medical education states the problem this way (3):

> Socialization processes prepare professionals for autonomy, but do not build in mechanisms for colleague control, much less any tolerance of attempts by outsiders to control activities over which professionals claim expertise.

The retreat environment raises expectations in its participants that may be new and unfamiliar to them. Thus, even though intimate group interaction and close group scrutiny are designed to support self-determined growth, they can be intrusive, particularly compared with the environment of the usual practice community, where people adjust their professional distance from colleagues and peers to suit their individual needs. "Retreating" may thus be a threat to the kind of familiar and complete professional autonomy that is reinforced at every turn in daily clinical practice.

Learning retreats may also seem unsatisfactory to potential participants in the way they deal with uncertainty. (See Chapter 25, A Touch of Cancer.) Clinical medicine is full of uncertainties: ambiguous data, incomplete information, unusual presentations, atypical therapeutic responses. One important way of dealing with uncertainty is that of turning to authorities: those with more experience, more expertise, more charisma, or public acceptance and recognition (4,5). The search for authoritative opinion surfaces in all CME programs. Learners are always hungry to know: "How do the experts see this problem? How do they think about it? How do they handle it?" (which, in light of learners' highly developed autonomy needs, also seems paradoxical—but then, people are not all of a piece). Content experts play an important role in learning retreats, but compared with conventional CME, their role is very much a secondary one. The emphasis in retreats is on self-initiated learning with the help of colleagues and, to a lesser degree, facilitators. This is an arrangement that may not satisfy the powerful need for authoritative opinion.

Learning retreats, then, are an attractive and powerful CME option, close perhaps to an educational ideal, and as such, deserve much wider use. But despite their many attractions, retreats suffer the way all ideal programs do when they come up against complex realities. The search for ideal CME is not yet over.

REFERENCES

1. **Fox RD, Mazmanian PE, Putnam RW.** Changing and Learning in the Lives of Physicians. New York: Praeger; 1989.
2. **Deci EL, Valelrand RJ, Pelletier LG, Ryan RM.** Motivation and education: the self-determination perspective. Educational Psychologist. 1991;26:325-46.
3. **Bucher R, Stelling JG.** Becoming Professional. Sage Library of Social Research. Vol. 46. London: Sage Publications; 1977:285.
4. **Light D Jr.** Uncertainty and control in professional training. J Health Soc Behav. 1979;20:310-22.
5. **Bosk C.** Forgive and Remember: Managing Medical Failure. Chicago: University of Chicago Press; 1979.

CHAPTER 16

Why Is Teaching Valued Less Than Research?

Those who can, do;
Those who can't, teach;
Those who can't teach, teach teachers.

ANONYMOUS

The purest coin of the academic realm is new knowledge, and finding new knowledge, of course, requires original research. Teaching, by way of contrast, is a debased intellectual currency in the academic marketplace; nobody gets promoted on the academic track for their teaching, at least not solely for teaching. Moreover, it is often the younger faculty, those least able to protect their time, who are tasked with the lion's share of teaching duties. Their seniors have earned the "right" to be free of such distractions and can devote themselves to research. What lies behind this strange view of the world?

The obvious explanation is that there is more money for research, and academic rewards go where the money is (Sutton's rule). But this explanation is too facile, really no explanation at all, since it doesn't explain why there is so much more money for research than for teaching in the first place. (We are talking here about teaching above the high school level. Prebaccalaureate education, of course, receives both public and private support, for many social and political reasons, although the teachers in that part of the education system are notoriously underpaid.) The answer has to lie deeper, closer to the reason why the creation of new knowledge, rather than the teaching of students, is considered the principal purpose of universities. It is therefore a matter of underlying values, not money. The question then becomes "what drives these underlying values?" Explanations are not difficult to find:

- Teaching does not create a tangible, deliverable product; it is more a process. The results of research, by contrast, can be seen, touched, counted, even weighed.

- Excellence in teaching is a local intellectual currency: There is no national standard, and hence it cannot be easily transported to new institutions or exchanged in new academic markets. Research is judged nationally and internationally and by widely shared standards.

- Henry Adams commented that "a teacher affects eternity." He added, optimistically, that "[a teacher] can never tell where his influence stops"; the obvious emphasis here is on the never-ending influence of teachers. But a wistful second meaning slipped through as well: It is hard for teachers to know what their impact has been. Thus, teaching excellence is not seen as leaving a lasting imprint; its effect on students quickly blends in with other influences, is soon damped out. Research excellence becomes a matter of unequivocal, individual public record that resonates for a long time; the best research is cited and indexed for decades, centuries, even millennia. Not surprisingly, authorship is a critical issue in research, a much sought-after but closely guarded prerogative.

- Everyone teaches at least some of the time. Parents teach children; brothers, sisters, and friends teach each other. It is only a small step, therefore, to the belief that anyone can teach and, beyond that, the belief that anyone can teach well. And, after all, everyone learns; indeed some people seem to be largely self-taught, which leads ultimately to the suspicion, deep down, that teachers may not be necessary at all. Research, in contrast—at least research in the formal, rigorous, scholarly sense—is not part of everyone's experience, of everyday life. Much of it is counterintuitive, a struggle against the tyranny of conventional wisdom, particular passions, personal biases. Research, therefore, belongs to the chosen few, the highly trained elite.

- Teaching is by its very nature a shared undertaking. Indeed, the best teachers are often known by their ability to remain very much in the background. Research, while often requiring enormous effort and great sacrifice, and often benefiting the many, is essentially focused on one person, the researcher, toiling alone in his or her world of new truths.

Each of these explanations has the ring of truth, but even taken together, they fail to explain convincingly the extraordinary hold of research over the values and the reward systems of academe. The clue to the mystery may lie, as it often does, in the extremes, both the bad and the good.

On the bad side, take the matter of violation of standards. In the case of research, such a violation—research fraud—is an extremely serious offense; it can and often does permanently damage a researcher's career. Teachers, like researchers, can be weak or uninspired and, like researchers, can falsify credentials or otherwise behave unethically. But while researchers are held rigidly and directly accountable for what they put forth, teachers are not. "Teaching fraud" is a nonissue; it is doubtful if the concept even exists, at least in any sense like that in which the concept of fraud is applied in research. This curious discrepancy is linked to the perception of research as a search for truth. That is, those who come close to something as powerful as truth are held in awe; researchers are expected, in return, to hold to an uncompromising standard, and hence violators fall rapidly from grace. Teachers, in contrast, are seen as messengers, at one remove from truth; they stand in relation to researchers in much the same way that critics do to creative artists, or performers to playwrights and composers: as recipients of derivative power.

Looked at from the positive side, the greatest researchers are heroes. Among their ranks are the Nobel laureates, endowed with magisterial power and authority. And then, greatest among the teachers there is . . . Mr. Chips? Beloved and appreciated, to be sure, but not particularly respected. Heroism takes many forms: raw strength and courage, defense of the weak, self-sacrifice. But heroism's most enduring expression lies in exploration of the unknown—the voyages of the starship *Enterprise*. Mission: "To boldly go where no one has gone before . . . " Explorers find new places, settlers follow in their footsteps; researchers find new knowledge, teachers teach what researchers have discovered, what is already known. Research is action, creation; teaching is re-action, re-creation.

Or so goes the conventional wisdom. However, on closer inspection of what really happens in teaching and research, the distinction between the two breaks down. Think of it this way: When, through good teaching, a student understands a truth he or she didn't understand before, that knowledge is just as new to the student as the discovery of a new truth through research is to the researcher and to the world at large. The principal difference is that, in the student's case the "new" knowledge is already known to many other people, while the researcher's "new" knowledge must be new to all of human thinking, otherwise it's not a true discovery. Since researcher-created newness is seen as heroic, while teacher-created newness is not, it is precisely this element of newness to the human race that must account for the enormous value placed on research. How else can we explain why the race for discovery, the struggle for priority, is so intense, so uncompromising in research (1)?

In fact, a great many "new" research discoveries later turn out to be rediscoveries, the original having been overlooked or forgotten. (Ironically, prior discovery often doesn't seem to reduce the credit assigned to the later researcher, as long as the rediscovery was truly arrived at independently.) Looking even further, the steps in the cyclic process by which researchers generate new knowledge—defining a problem, asking the right questions, getting the answers (data), portraying and interpreting the results, which define the next problem—map exactly onto the steps in the process by which students acquire new knowledge (i.e., new to them), at least when they acquire it through experiential learning—concrete experience, reflective observation on that experience, abstract conceptualization, followed by active experimentation in the next experience (2). (See Chapter 24, the Right Hand of Claude.) In most of the ways that matter, then, both the process and the product of teaching are identical to those of research. In light of this, how can we say that the student's new knowledge is any less important than that of the researchers? And how can we say that teachers who bring forth new knowledge in their students deserve any less credit than their knowledge-delivering counterparts in research?

Alas for teaching, the intrinsically equivalent value of these two forms of new knowledge has been caught up in and largely obscured by the ubiquitous struggle for control, for power. Teaching is by its very nature a shared enterprise; hence it has trouble arrogating power to itself in the same way that research can. The disparities run throughout the worlds of teaching and research: even the standard distribution systems for the work of researchers (e.g., publication) vastly outweigh those available to teachers (e.g., the classroom). Indeed, when teaching becomes highly efficient and effective, it paradoxically becomes suspect.

The psychiatrist Thomas Szasz clearly, if somewhat bitterly, articulated this curious discordance between power and teaching:

> We can conclude that—the psychology of human relationships being what it is—in adult education there is an inverse relationship between "power" and "learning." Only the "weak" can teach. If the teacher comes into too much power, he ceases to be a "teacher" and becomes instead a religious or political (or other "group") "leader."

Is there reason to expect that the balance of power in academe between research and teaching can be shifted? And should it be shifted? There are certainly those who feel the present balance is just where it ought to be. Perhaps that shift will happen, although probably not in our lifetime. Until it does, those on the teaching side would do well to remember that power corrupts, and that, in the greater scheme of things, the new knowledge created in students' minds through the efforts of teachers is not distinguishable from the new knowledge created by researchers.

REFERENCES

1. **Watson JD.** The Double Helix: A Personal Account of the Discovery of the Structure of DNA. New York: Atheneum; 1968.
2. **Kolb DA.** Experiential Learning. Experience as the Source of Learning and Development. Englewood Cliffs, NJ: PTR Prentice Hall; 1984:33.

CHAPTER 17

Mystery, Murder, and Medicine

~

Reading the Clues

Murder mysteries and medicine have a great deal in common. The most obvious affinity lies in the similarity between detection and diagnosis: observing keenly, asking the right questions, seeing patterns. Sherlock Holmes's pronouncement, "When you have eliminated the impossible, whatever remains, *however improbable, must be the truth*" (from *The Sign of Four*, published in 1890) eloquently articulates the kind of hypotheco-deductive reasoning used by both doctors and detectives (1). It is arguably the example medical writers quote most often (some would say too often) in affirming this special shared way of thinking. And this mutual fascination with puzzling things out turns up in mystery fiction again and again, as in a 1928 Dorothy Sayers story involving her aristocratic detective, Lord Peter Wimsey (2):

> "It must be fascinatin', diagnosin' things," said Peter thoughtfully. "How d'you do it? I mean, is there a regular set of symptoms for each disease, like callin' a club to show you want your partner to go no trumps? You don't just say: 'This fellow's got a pimple on his nose, therefore he has fatty degeneration of the heart—"
>
> "I hope not," said the doctor dryly.
>
> "Or is it more like gettin' a clue to a crime?" went on Peter. "You see somethin'—a room, or a body, say, all knocked about anyhow, and there's a damn sight of symptoms of somethin' wrong, and you've got just to pick out the ones that tell the story?"
>
> "That's more like it," said Dr. Hartman.

But a link at the level of diagnosis and detection is just the beginning; the closer you look, the more intimate and intricate the relationship becomes. The first clue comes from the intriguing observation that so many (presumably) normal, decent people are dedicated murder mystery fans. Question: Why are people so endlessly fascinated by tales of killing and blood and mayhem? Asked to explain this baffling loyalty, aficionados of the genre answer without hesitation:

- Murder is the ultimate creator of disorder—anxiety, terror, disruption.
- Bringing the perpetrator of a murder to justice is deeply satisfying because it restores order.   Q.E.D.

Or, in Sayers's words (3)

> The desire of being persuaded that all human experience may be presented in terms of a problem having a predictable, final, complete and sole possible solution accounts, to a great extent, for the late extraordinary popularity of detective fiction.

The outlines of another parallel between medicine and murder mystery now begin to take shape, since

- Even apart from its occasional role as a killer, disease is also a notorious perpetrator of anxiety, disruption, and disorder in patients' bodies and in their lives. (Recall that *dis-order* is a principal synonym for disease.)
- Restoring order means making things whole again; indeed, the verb "to heal" comes from a root meaning "to make whole."   Q.E.D.

Detectives and doctors, then, are more than solvers of puzzles: Both are also restorers of order, particularly in the face of violence done to the body. So far, so good. But there's violence and there's violence, and the reaction varies accordingly. The violence of boxing, hockey, and other sports, for example, brings rewards—huge crowds and equally huge salaries; even killing on the battlefield brings honor. But murder, in contrast, is universally feared and despised, an abominable, shameful, and degraded act, worthy of the worst punishments imaginable, including death. Question: Why the difference? Here language provides the clue, for the word murder originally (4)

> denoted *secret* murder, which in Germanic antiquity was alone regarded (in the modern sense) a crime, open homicide being regarded a private wrong calling for blood-revenge or compensation.

It is secrecy, then, that makes the violence of murder so heinous: secret acts are cowardly, guilty acts; a murderer, being anonymous, is not an individual and is therefore less than human; and the devil you don't know is always more threatening than the devil you know. By the same token, detection—finding out "who dunnit"—is ultimately a moral act, since it converts the unknown, a faceless creature who cannot be called to account, into the known, a flesh-and-blood killer now answerable for his or her crime. A third, most subtle link to medicine is thus revealed. For while disease is not murder, undiagnosed illness shares some of murder's immoral qualities: threatening, or shameful, or degrading exactly *because* the "perpetrator" is secret (5).

From this perspective, diagnosis in medicine takes on something of the same moral quality as detection in murder mysteries; by bringing the causal agent into the light, both neutralize the malevolent, guilty quality associated with unknown causes. The way this works is itself a bit mysterious, but both diagnosis and detection depend for their effect on at least three major acts: naming, predicting, and explaining. (Note that while some detectives resort in the course of their work to selective, "surgical" violence, the act of detection is at its core an act of nonviolence, of thinking.) The most immediate goal in both detection and diagnosis is, of course, to identify specifically *who* (or *what*) is responsible for the violence—to give him (or it) a *name*: the personal identity of the murderer, or the diagnostic entity responsible for the patient's distress, as the case may be. By giving form to the formless, naming itself carries great power, for better or for worse. Recall the old apocryphal story about the patient who was so relieved when his doctor told him that his sore tongue was "glossitis." And think of the benefits and risks that result when real patients are labeled with medical diagnoses (6,7).

But naming, general or specific, does more than bring tangible things out of the void. The story is told that students of the great Swedish taxonomist Linnaeus played a practical joke by hanging a huge moosehead over the old master's bed at night while he was asleep. When they woke him, he glanced up at the moosehead and said, "Antlers, grinding teeth—herbivore; won't bite me," and promptly went back to sleep. Naming lets you classify, and classification lets you predict what will happen.

But rational, effective intervention, whether it is bringing a murderer to justice or successfully treating pulmonary edema, ultimately demands more than classification; it requires explanation. For the homicide detective, explanation equals learning the means, motive, and opportunity of a murderer; for the doctor, it equals understanding the etiology, anatomy, and pathophysiology of a disease—and, in both detection and medicine, it is here that science enters the picture. It can hardly be an accident, after all, that Arthur Conan Doyle, himself a physician, created the modern genre of mystery fiction just at the time scientific thinking had begun seriously to influence medicine. (See Chapter 2, Information and Education.)

Now there is little doubt that, on balance, science has transformed both crime detection and medical diagnosis for the better. At the same time, unfortunately, the rational, scientific approach used in both detective fiction and diagnosis is a source of serious difficulty, giving rise to the distortions described by Dorothy Sayers in her extraordinary essay, "Problem Picture" (2). Detective fiction writers, she notes, are bound by a rigid canon of "the mathematical or detective problem," namely, that the detective problem is

1. Always soluble (i.e., constructed for the express purpose of being solved)
2. Completely soluble (i.e., no loose ends)
3. Solved in the same terms in which it is set (i.e., without stepping outside its terms of reference), and
4. Finite (i.e., when it is solved, there is an end of it).

But careless use of the words *problem* and *solution* in medicine in the same way they are used in detective fiction distorts the thinking about real diseases of real patients, because real disorders of real patients don't fit into the narrow, artificial mold of detective fiction. As she puts it (2):

> We continue to hug the delusion that all ill-health is caused by some single, definite disease, for which there ought to be a single, definite and complete cure without unfortunate after-effects. We think of our illness as a kind of cross-word *of which the answer is known to somebody*: the complete solution must be *there*, somewhere; it is the doctor's business to discover and apply it.

But, Sayers continues, the physician is not solving a crossword puzzle.

> He is performing a delicate, adventurous, and experimental creative act, of which the patient's body is the material, and to which the creative cooperation of the patient's will is necessary. He is not rediscovering a state of health, temporarily obscured; he is remaking it, or rather, helping it to remake itself.

The lure of medical diagnosis is powerful, largely, it appears, because of the expectation that diagnosing diseases will be like solving the mathematics-like puzzles of detective fiction. Real-life diagnostic work, unfortunately, rarely conforms to that unrealistic expectation, which probably explains many of its frustrations (8). The lesson here, then, is that medicine is not a candidate for the "Detection Club," where membership is contingent on a willingness never to violate the defined terms of the problem. Medicine, like most of real life, usually sets its problems in terms that *must* be violated if they are to be dealt with at all.

Final question: Do homicide detectives like to read murder mysteries?

REFERENCES

1. **Elstein AS, Shulman LS, Sprafka SA.** Medical Problem Solving: An Analysis of Clinical Reasoning. Cambridge, MA: Harvard University Press; 1978.
2. **Sayers DL.** The vindictive story of the footsteps that ran. In: Lord Peter Views the Body. New York: Avon Books; 1969:135.
3. **Sayers DL.** Problem Picture. In: The Mind of the Maker. New York: Harper & Row; 1987.
4. **Oxford English Dictionary.** [The Compact Edition] Complete Text Reproduced Micrographically. New York: Oxford University Press; 1971:1877.
5. **Sontag S.** Illness as Metaphor. New York: Farrar, Straus and Giroux; 1978.
6. **Ward BW, Wu WC, Richter JE, Hackshaw BT, Castell DO.** Long-term follow-up of symptomatic status of patients with non-cardiac chest pain: is diagnosis of esophageal etiology helpful? Am J Gastroenterol. 1987;82:215-8.
7. **Haynes RB, Sackett DL, Taylor DW, Gibson ES, Johnson AL.** Increased absenteeism from work after detection and labeling of hypertension patients. N Engl J Med. 1978;299:741-3.
8. **Glenn ML.** On Diagnosis: A Systemic Approach. New York: Brunner/Mazel; 1984.

CHAPTER 18

Who Has Seen a Blood Sugar?

❧

The Shaping of the Invisible World

*I*n my years as a clinical diabetologist, my patients' blood sugars were very real to me. Individual blood sugar numbers on a lab slip, or in a patient's notebook, were almost tangible; a graphic display of sugars over time drawn out for a patient was even more powerfully vivid for us both.

Yet one day I realized that, despite my intimacy with blood sugars, I had never actually seen one. I had obviously seen plenty of blood; I had certainly seen plenty of sugar. But the *level of sugar in someone's blood?* No. For all its conceptual power, medical utility, psychological meaning—for all its reality—I'd never laid eyes on it.

How can something invisible be so real? Perhaps that isn't such a mystery when you consider that the very essence of medical education is to create those very intangibles, the mental models of anatomical structure, physiological function, and pathophysiological dislocations. The models laboriously are built up in students' minds, starting with premedical study and continuing right on through residency, fact by fact, concept by concept, one on top of the other; they are woven together into a truly extraordinary conceptual structure, a whole virtual world. Over time, that world becomes so real, so tangible, that once we have entered it, we never quite leave it. It takes on the quality of *cyberspace,* the concept originally created by author William Gibson to describe what people interface *with* when they enter an electronic "information highway," a kind of super-real merging of inner mind with external constructs (1). (Others have described cyberspace as "the place where your long-distance telephone conversation *really* takes place" or "the place where the bank *really* keeps your money.")

From the foot of the bed, Hippocrates saw a person with Hippocratic facies. In our mind's eye, we see inside that person a mitral valve, covered with septic excrescences; our mental "zoom lens" then moves down into an image of purple gram-positive bugs in pink fibrin; back out to the telltale shapes on the trans-esophageal echo; and on to the image of halos around antibiotic disks in a petri dish. Our ability to give shape to the invisible by entering medical cyberspace (or perhaps more accurately, biomedical cyberspace) is a large part of what gives us our power, our leverage over disease. We guard it jealously, as we should. Patients, families, and nonphysicians generally can't enter it—or, at most, can only penetrate the margins.

The immediacy of medical cyberspace makes even more sense in light of Seymour Papert's more general Piagetian view of learning (2). Papert describes his discovery, at age two, of automobile gears:

> It was, of course, many years later before I understood how gears work; but once I did, playing with gears became a favorite pastime. I loved rotating circular objects against one another in gearlike motions.

His fascination with gears served over time as the basis for both his intellectual grasp of mathematical ideas and his abiding passion for the discipline of mathematics, literally through a kinesthetic appreciation of the subject. ("You can be the gear, you can understand how it turns by projecting yourself into its place and turning with it.")

From these experiences and his work with children programming computers, Papert (2) concludes that

> What an individual can learn, and how he learns it, depends on what models he has available. This raises, recursively, the question of how he learned these models. Thus, the "laws of learning" must be about how intellectual structures grow out of one another and about how, in the process, they acquire both logical and emotional form.

Papert's view finds echoes in many places, from Ayn Rand's general comment that "mankind tends to drift toward the primacy of consciousness, the supremacy of thought," to the recent specific suggestion that clinical expertise in medicine "is not so much a matter of superior reasoning skills or in-depth knowledge of pathophysiological states as it is based on *cognitive structures* that describe the features of prototypical or even actual patients" (3; emphasis added)—"illness scripts" in the authors' terminology.

Despite their intense reality, medical concepts aren't easy to represent outside your head. Of course, words are the principal "left brain" medium for capturing them. But imaging techniques play an increasing (and increasingly expensive) role as "right brain" representations of medical disease models; and diagrams are often the only way to see intricate pathophysiological relationships. Curiously, medical decision logic, which lies at the heart of clinical medicine, has been among the most difficult dimensions of the invisible to visualize, and indeed has gone largely unrepresented in medical cyberspace. More recently, however, an "imaging technique for visualizing medical logic," the discipline of medical decision analysis, has at last come along (4).

The existence of medical mental models—medical cyberspace— seems as indispensable as it is indisputable. Unfortunately, in creating, transmitting, and using these models, we have struck a Faustian bargain, trading a piece of our souls in exchange for the power of knowledge. For we seem to have created a situation in which *medical cyberspace seems more real to us than the sick patient in the bed.* What are the consequences of this bargain?

To begin with, there is the gallows humor about the patient who dies with her electrolytes in perfect order ("she was euboxic"—an ironic expression that refers to the little boxes in the medical record where electrolyte values are recorded). This says to us that it doesn't matter so much what happened to the patient in the bed, as long as the more real concept, the electrolytes (which, incidentally, no one has ever actually seen any more than they've seen a blood sugar), were "cured." Then there are the not-so-funny references to "the ulcer in room 32," ironic, again, because the concept is more real than the live patient.

Is it any wonder, then, that clinical teaching now happens mostly in the conference room rather than at the bedside? The visible, but *less real,* patient in the bed becomes something of a hindrance; the patient gets in the way of the *more real* discussion, the one about the invisible *concepts.* Can it be an accident that autopsy rates continue to drop? It is increasingly difficult, it seems, to extract much conceptually useful material out of the intensely visible autopsy. Is it such a mystery that we order lab test after lab test, then test again? Mental models of a patient's disease states may be intensely real, but they are, after all, a shadowy, flickering reality that easily slips away. It is a reality that can never be quite clear enough, that needs continuous reinforcing with tangible outward representations we can cling to: the images, the numbers.

Even psychiatry, the medical discipline closest to the human side of patients' lives, has been charged with trying too hard to fit the person's life situation, Procrustes-like, into pre-formed mental models. Thus (5),

> First-year medical students often obtain textured and subtle autobiographical accounts from patients and offer them to others with enthusiasm and pleasure, whereas fourth-year students or house officers are apt to present cryptic, dryly condensed, and, yes, all too "structured" presentations, full of abbreviations, not to mention medical or psychiatric jargon . . . . It is not the rare patient who approaches a second doctor with the plea that he or she wasn't heard, that the first physician had his or her mind made up from the start of a consultation and went ahead accordingly with a diagnostic and therapeutic regimen.

It is probably also true that acute care hospitals, the current venue for most clinical teaching, reinforce the reality of the present, self-contained version of medical cyberspace. Biomedical concepts, images, and numbers are more urgently needed in dealing with the sicker patients and more complicated disease situations in hospitals than with the more stable patients outside them. And hospitalized patients often lack long-standing relationships with their caregivers, making it even harder for the staff to appreciate the reality of the sick person himself or herself relative to the reality of the illness script in their heads.

Invisible forces, particularly the "forces of nature," are among the oldest and most compelling of human concerns. The theologian Elaine Pagels reflects (6)

> on the ways that various religious traditions give shape to the invisible world, and how our imaginative perceptions of what is invisible relate to the ways we respond to the people around us, to events, and to the natural world.

As she points out, people in the ancient Western world assumed that the universe was inhabited by invisible beings whose presence impinged upon the visible world and its inhabitants, an assumption that carries widespread force even today, particularly in connection with misfortune, disease, and loss. Medicine shares with religion, then, the ability to give substance to the invisible world, which undoubtedly accounts in large measure for their intimate relationship over the centuries. The cyberspace universe of scientific medicine differs, to be sure, from an animist or monotheistic moral universe, but all such universes are concerned with explaining, rationalizing, and ultimately controlling the unpredicted, and unpredictable, disruptions of human life.

The lure of medical cyberspace is very powerful. The poet Christina

Rossetti may have touched on something more fundamental than she realized when she wrote her seemingly artless verse for children (7):

> Who has seen the wind?
> Neither you nor I;
> But when the trees bow down their heads
> The wind is passing by.

REFERENCES

1. **Gibson W.** Neuromancer. New York: Ace Books, Berkeley Publishing Co.; 1984.
2. **Papert S.** Mindstorms. Children, Computers, and Powerful Ideas. New York: Basic Books; 1980.
3. **Schmidt HG, Norman GR, Boshuizen HP.** A cognitive perspective on medical expertise: theory and implications. Acad Med. 1990;65:611-21.
4. **Davidoff F.** Decision analysis: an imaging technique for visualizing medical logic. In: Nobel J, ed. Textbook of General Medicine and Primary Care. Boston: Little, Brown; 1988:27–34.
5. **Coles R.** The Call of Stories. Teaching and the Moral Imagination. Boston: Houghton Mifflin; 1989.
6. **Pagels E.** The Origin of Satan. New York: Random House; 1995.
7. **Rossetti C.** Who has seen the wind? In: The Golden Journey. Poems for Young People. Compiled by Bogan L, Smith WJ. Chicago: Reilly & Lee; 1965:33.

CHAPTER *19*

Manners

Getting the Meta-Message

Thingis somtyme alowed is now repreuid.

CAXTON'S BOOK OF CURTEYSE

(Fifteenth Century)

When things go awry in the care of patients, the problem is commonly diagnosed as "communication failure," particularly when it occurs during patient referral or consultation. To be sure, referring physicians don't always provide all the clinical information they should, or formulate their questions clearly, or make their expectations clear about responsibility for care. And consultants not infrequently fail to answer the referring doctor's question, or provide too much, or too little, or irrelevant information. And lack of information, or inexact information, or wrong information clearly can and does create all kinds of havoc with the quality of care.

The usual therapy for "bad communication disease" therefore is the well-intentioned advice that those involved should be more complete, more accurate, more direct in the future. After all, the thinking goes, how can the care process work unless the information available is timely, clear, complete? But despite the obvious "rightness" of this reasoning and the advice that flows from it, "bad communication disease" is quite difficult to treat, and the results of the usual therapeutic approach are frequently not encouraging.

The difficulty with the communication-focused approach may be that communication failure is not the "disease" at all, but a "symptom," more like fever, say, than like subacute bacterial endocarditis. Telling people who have messed up a communication to remember to do it better next time may therefore be like trying to treat SBE by giving acetaminophen to bring the fever down. In fact, the correct underlying diagnosis for the problem underlying the symptom of communication failure may be something altogether different—namely, discourtesy, disrespect, or just plain rudeness. Discourtesy is, of course, defined partly by the person affected by it, which immediately raises the question of whom a referring physician or a consultant is being discourteous *to* when he or she communicates badly. The answer would seem to be *both* to the other physician *and* to the patient. Not to put too fine a point on it, it is just plain rude to the consultant, and to the patient, to fail to prepare and share the right information.

Formulating the problem of communication failure in terms of discourtesy shifts the frame of reference entirely, from that of information transfer to that of *manners*. But the manners we are talking about here are not things like using the correct fork at dinner or crooking your pinkie when you drink tea: those are affectations more than manners. We are talking about something much more fundamental, a critical social force that has been called by many names, including *civility* and *civilization* and *culture*, and whose importance (at least in European history) has been described as nothing less than "the self-consciousness of the West" (1).

In essence, manners serve two main social purposes: control of people's own impulses, and recognition of, or consideration for, other people's feelings and situations. Manners in this sense extend back at least as far as written history itself, as in this bit of Viking advice on restraint in conversation written in about 800 AD (2):

> Much nonsense
> a man utters
> who talks without tiring.
> A ready tongue
> unrestrained
> brings bad reward.

Not surprisingly, much of the early writing on manners was preoccupied with basic functions such as eating, talking, spitting, blowing one's nose, passing gas, aggressiveness, and behavior toward the opposite sex. What is considered civilized behavior has evolved, sometimes slowly, sometimes rather abruptly. The changes over time in acceptable or desirable behavior have generally been in the direction suggested by the quotation given at the beginning of this chapter, namely, "Things that were once allowed are now reproved." Thus, the evolution of manners over time has reflected a progressive metamorphosis of what originally were direct, active ways of dealing with other people, often aggressively and at their expense, into passive, more ordered pleasures, such as spectator sports, or parades, or theater—that is, the "mere" pleasures of the eye (1). Manners have also moved generally in the direction of a decreased threshold of embarrassment about things done publicly, and the concerns of manners have extended progressively outward from the biological to the social aspects of human affairs, including social class, status, and group identity.

The anthropologist Gregory Bateson threw a different light on manners when he pointed out that any speech or behavior potentially carries two messages: its surface content, or direct message, and its symbolic content or "meta-message"—the "message beyond the message." (The interpretation of social meta-messages shades over into the more general discipline of "semiotics," the reading of signs.) To take an everyday example, a memo that says "Your boss has been promoted" gives you the specific knowledge that someone's position in the organization has changed—the memo's direct or surface content; but it also lets you know that someone in the organization thinks you matter enough to include you on the distribution list for the memo. Thus, the very fact of being sent the memo itself carries important symbolic meaning, a meta-message if you like, about who you are and where you stand; if you doubt this is true, just go talk to the people who weren't sent the memo. Or, to take a medical example, the important but unpleasant nursing task of cleaning up a fecally incontinent patient carries the surface content of: I am making you physically more comfortable. The meta-message, in contrast, is: I recognize that being incontinent is embarrassing, and by cleaning you up, I can give you back some of your dignity.

Manners, then, are meta-messages—speech and behaviors that carry symbolic, social meanings—which, in medicine as elsewhere, are often at least as important as the surface content, sometimes more so. The meta-message of manners is frequently quite nonspecific, like the custom of switching your knife from your right to your left hand to eat after you have cut up your food, which has been interpreted in a general way to mean "this is the way we do it in America, as opposed to the way they do it in Europe." But the very same behavior can carry a specific, pointed meta-message, as in certain Quaker communities in the United States, where a knife held in the right hand, when not being used to cut food, represents a weapon. The meta-message of manners is therefore determined as much by the receiver as by the sender, which means, of course, that misunderstandings arise when the sender doesn't know about the receiver's customary interpretation. Things obviously go more smoothly when the sender and the receiver both understand the meta-messages of certain manners in the same way.

Thus, a consultation note from an internist telling an anesthesiologist not to let the blood pressure go too low during surgery in a patient with coronary disease contains a message that on the face of it seems perfectly reasonable. But an anesthesiologist may well interpret such a note as dis- courteous—that is, carrying the meta-message that the internist doesn't recognize and respect the anesthesiologist's experience, intelligence, and good clinical judgment. Similar problems appear when referring physi- cians don't provide the appropriate clinical background to consultants, or when they don't formulate their questions clearly. Since the consultants then have to spend time chasing down the necessary information, it is easy for them to interpret the failure to receive information as meaning that referring doctors don't recognize the value of their (the consultants') time. The same kind of meta-message is sent in reverse when consultants don't report back promptly—or at all—to referring physicians. In this case, the failure to communicate the medical (surface) content is obvi- ously bad medicine on the grounds that being deprived of the surface (medical) content makes it hard for the referring doctors to make good clinical decisions. But what often troubles referring physicians most in this situation is the lack of courtesy implicit in the failure of consultants to report back, because that failure carries the meta-message that consul- tants don't respect the referring physicians and hence are ignoring them.

Mention of manners often evokes associations with gender, in the sense that mannerly behavior is thought of as "doing what your mother taught you." While the implications of any such inference extend far beyond this discussion, there is certainly evidence that men tend to be concerned more with formal rules (where the surface content matters, as in law, business, sports, government, the military) and less with the informal rules (the meta-messages, including manners, that express, shape, and govern per- sonal relationships), while for women, the priorities are, generally speaking, reversed. To the extent that women do focus more directly on the rules of interpersonal behavior, then, mothers may well play the greater role in socializing children with regard to manners. Medicine may also reflect these gender-linked perspectives, since medicine has, until recently, been indisputably dominated by men. Gender differences such as these might help explain a number of otherwise obscure aspects of medical culture—such as why communication failure is thought of in terms of formal rules (e.g., failure to provide clear, concise information to your consultants), rather than in terms of socially meaningful meta-messages (e.g., failure to treat your consultants courteously). (See Chapter 21, Bankers and Midwives.)

Manners may have also been pushed aside in medicine because of the "battlefield" metaphor that dominates the culture of hospitals. Thus, the work of hospitals is seen as the "war against disease"; doctors in hospitals come into contact with more dead bodies than practically anyone else in society other than soldiers (and undertakers); and hospitals are places where chains of command and other such military metaphors are commonplace. Hospitals are fast-moving, high-pressure places; places of life and death and blood and guts; places where, it seems, there is little room for niceties like civility and courtesy. And hospitals are almost exclusively the places where medical students and residents have been socialized for over 100 years.

There is a certain irony in all this. Where else, if not in medicine, should extreme civility be the rule? Being sick is distressing, disturbing, and horrifying enough when one is not being treated rudely by anybody. It is exactly when people are sickest that they most need respect and courtesy. And taking care of sick people is complicated, uncertain, and demanding enough for the caretakers without the added burden of discourtesy from anybody. It is exactly when doctors are most challenged that it is most important they treat each other with consideration.

Grace under pressure isn't bad as an explicit, major professional goal. And learning and teaching how to make the underlying diagnosis of "lack of courtesy" or sometimes even "just plain rudeness" correctly when it occurs, rather than simply pointing to the symptom of "communication failure," might be a refreshing and effective move toward improving the way we take care of patients, and the way we deal with each other in doing it.

REFERENCES

1. **Elias N.** The Civilizing Process. The History of Manners. New York: Urizen Books; 1978:3.
2. **Hávamál.** The Sayings of the Vikings. Translated by Björn Jónasson. Reykjavík, Iceland: Gudrún Publishing House; 1992.

CHAPTER 20

Quitting

~

May the Force Be with You

As she settled back into her chair, my neighbor at the table at a recent wedding reception table sheepishly explained her ten-minute absence: "I'm afraid I'm one of those people who just hasn't been able to quit cigarettes." Curiosity getting the better of me, I asked what it was about smoking that kept her doing it. "Oh," she said, "it's like your friend." Then, reflecting a little, she added emphatically, "It's like the best friend you ever had."

You want power, I'll show you power! Is it any wonder that no one, including a physician, is very effective in getting other people to quit smoking? What we understand about why people smoke and, thus, how we try to help patients to quit don't seem to come even close to the source of cigarettes' power over people's lives. Indeed, until recently, the explanatory model most widely used by physicians has been a rather simple one: "Patients choose to do it, so they could therefore just as easily choose not to if they tried." A stripped-down, slightly moralistic understanding like this has left us little choice about our role in getting patients to quit, other than telling them to "just say no" and why. While this approach works, it does so only 5 percent of the time or less. Clearly, there's room for improvement.

Fortunately, research done in the past decade has now given us a much richer understanding of the power of cigarette smoking. One key development, of course, is the unequivocal if belated recognition that nicotine is an addicting chemical, which has been accompanied by the development of new ways of thinking about how addiction works in general (1). Another is the recognition that the behavior change involved in quitting is itself a complex process involving specific stages, namely, precontemplation, contemplation, and preparation, followed by action, and, eventually, maintenance (2). The emergence of these new and rather pragmatic mental models has enabled the development of new and pragmatic therapies: thus, nicotine substitution and counseling programs designed specifically to move patients from one stage in the behavior change process to the next.

But for all their apparent rightness and good sense, these models still fall short of a fully satisfying explanation. For one thing, it is now clear that other compulsive behaviors such as gambling and running, where external chemicals are not used, can take on the qualities of true addiction. This observation alone suggests that it would be naive to depend too heavily on a biophysical explanation for the addicting quality of behaviors such as cigarette smoking, where external chemicals clearly do play a role. (Endorphins are sometimes invoked to explain non-chemical addictions, but this explanation ducks the issue of why some nonchemical-using behaviors are addicting while others aren't.) For another thing, while nicotine patches and tailored behavior-change therapies are more effective than simply urging patients to "just say no," they are still no match for the power of "the weed" (2). We are clearly going to need a considerably stronger counterforce than we have now if we are going to confront that power successfully. Moreover, in the face of a creature as devious, as subtle, as cunning as the cigarette, a crude or frontal approach is unlikely to work; what we need, rather, is an understanding so sophisticated, so deep, that we can outsmart the beast.

Part of that necessary deep understanding may be contained in the notion that "cigarettes are sublime." In his book by that name (3), Richard Klein writes that "warning smokers or neophytes of the dangers entices them more powerfully to the edge of the abyss, where, like travelers in a Swiss landscape, they can be thrilled by the subtle grandeur of the perspectives on mortality opened by the little terrors in every puff. Cigarettes are bad. That is why they are [seen as] good—not good, not beautiful, but sublime." Here Klein clearly uses the word "sublime" not in its stripped down, twentieth century meaning of "supreme" or "noble," but pointedly in its dark, nineteenth century sense of what Kant called "a negative pleasure." Paintings from the last century frequently gloried in representing the sublime: the image of towering clouds from an onrushing storm contrasted with the tiny, vulnerable human figures in a peaceable landscape, for example.

Human fascination with negative pleasures seems never to diminish, finding gross, outward latter-day expression in everything from driving too fast to rock climbing and bungee-jumping. But the sublime is also part of the lure of other more subtle and seductive experiences, however noxious, dangerous, or terrifying they may be—experiences, such as smoking cigarettes, that also make people feel fully "alive," connected to the great forces in the universe. Tobacco qualifies as a negative pleasure on all counts. Long before its specific health risks were identified, tobacco was widely seen as a threat, probably because it was so clearly mind altering and so addicting. And long before they start the habit, people today know perfectly well that smoking is a noxious and, ultimately, dangerous thing to do. Why otherwise the warning label on the cigarette package? Why otherwise the place of smoking among the "forbidden" experiences for children?

Admittedly, nowadays, in a culture awash with sound-bite explanation and refined-sugar gratification, it is a little tough to come to grips with an explanatory model as mysterious as the conundrum of "the sublime." However, once you deal with it (in the parlance of the day), it's not hard to see the many and various faces of the sublime in cigarette smoking. In his essay (written in part to help him quit), Klein reflects with hyperbolic relish on these many faces (3). Thus: smoking is a clock, each cigarette marking out the inexorable passage of time; for some people, cigarette smoking becomes the ultimate, the most defiant way to waste time, even the principal emblem of useless but pure "art for art's sake"; then there is the special sublime significance of cigarette smoking for women (independence, choice, toughness), and for men (the soldier's friend, more precious in war, at times, than food; and the various forms of macho, from Bogart's incessant smoking in "Casablanca," to the insidious adolescent appeal of the Marlboro man).

One particularly telling, and startling, aspect of the sublime in smoking is "quitting as a way of life." Zeno, the protagonist of a 1920s novel by the Italian author Italo Svevo, devotes his entire life to smoking and, as Klein tells us, much of it to quitting. Quitting does two things for Zeno: first, it makes him feel heroic. The problem is that while the resolution to quit lends him a kind of nobility, he also realizes that if he *actually* quit he would immediately lose this source of his self-esteem. Second, the last cigarette always takes on a particularly intense flavor for Zeno, both from the feeling of victory over himself and from the poignancy of the impending loss. The rewards of quitting themselves become so intense they prevent him from quitting; he goes on endlessly quitting, therefore, smoking one "final" cigarette after another.

The prospects of quitting for someone like Zeno, locked in the labyrinth of smoking, seem pretty dim. But, surprisingly, he does quit, and does so in a Houdini-like fashion that reaffirms the critical importance of patient autonomy in this decision (4). Thus, quitting becomes possible for Zeno only when he realizes that life itself is unhealthy; indeed, that unlike many other "diseases," life itself is always mortal. When he finally comes to look at his situation this way, Zeno realizes smoking is simply one way of living and no worse for his health than most other ways. And once he decides he is just as healthy if he does smoke as if he doesn't, he can stop responding to external pressures, including from his doctors, to "be healthy." This means he no longer has to continue making resolutions to quit, which at last allows him to quit, since quitting is now an autonomous, free choice rather than one imposed from outside.

This is, after all, fiction, and not all patients have Zeno's philosophical turn of mind. But Zeno's paradox does bring to the surface an important potential trap when dealing with the sublime. That is, those—like Zeno's doctors, as well as Mark Twain's fictional Aunt Mary (4)—who go up against smoking as crusaders risk taking on the functions of the patient's own conscience, thus allowing patients to say, in effect, "Now it's my doctor, not me, who wants me to stop this filthy, dangerous habit, and thank goodness for that. As long as my doctor isn't watching I don't have to worry about it." Posing, at the appropriate times, three deceptively simple questions to patients who smoke: "What do you understand about the health consequences of smoking?", "Are you ready to quit?", and "What would it take for you to stop smoking?" may help avoid this unwitting collusion between the patient's physician and the patient's conscience. By using these questions, doctors let patients know that they are staying with the problem and, at the same time, gently but firmly move the decision to quit back to the smoker.

Understanding and applying the complex "pathophysiology of the sublime" and the role of autonomy in behavior change may not be medicine exactly as we've known and loved it, taught and learned it, over the years. But to the extent that these sophisticated principles apply, they may be at least as powerful in the management of smoking and the induction of quitting as, say, the physiology of myocardial contraction and the pharmacology of angiotensin-converting enzyme inhibitors are in the management of congestive failure—and from many points of view, at least as important.

REFERENCES

1. **Hyman SE.** A man with alcoholism and HIV infection. JAMA. 1995;274:837-43.
2. **Rollnick S, Kinnersley P, Stott N.** Methods of helping patients with behaviour change. BMJ. 1993;307:188-90.
3. **Klein R.** Cigarettes are Sublime. Durham, NC: Duke University Press; 1993.
4. **Williams GC, Quill TE, Deci EL, Ryan RM.** "The facts concerning the recent carnival of *smoking* in Connecticut" *and elsewhere.* Ann Intern Med. 1991;115:59-63.

PART THREE

SYMBIOSIS

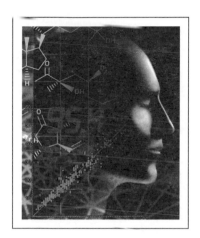

CHAPTER 21

Bankers and Midwives

Reflections on Education and Training

*T*he presenter of a seminar at the Artificial Intelligence Laboratory at MIT in the early 1980s said "You can't teach somebody something they don't already almost know." This Zen-like reflection came back recently as I read "Women's Ways of Knowing," a study based on hundreds of hours of interviews that provides an important perspective on the understandings women achieve, the voices they develop, and the ways these come about (1). The authors also examine the educational implications of this developmental process, implications that apply to men and women alike.

The aphorism from MIT implies that hosts of partly formed conceptual "infants" exist within every learner, just waiting to be "raised." Accordingly, teaching consists of nurturing, guiding, disciplining these young mental creatures, seeing to it that they grow into mature, adult knowledge. The metaphor evokes the very root of the word "educate," which the Oxford English Dictionary tells us is the Latin word "educare," to raise children.

Contrast these notions of teaching and learning with the "banking" model of education described in "Women's Ways of Knowing." In the banking model, which the authors argue developed in a male-dominated academic universe and in their view still makes up most of traditional education, faculty work out of sight to "mint" the material for their books and lectures, then bring it forth to "deposit" in students' minds like money in a savings account. The banking model is particularly germane to medical education in light of their assertions that "the problem is especially acute with respect to science," that "science is usually taught by males" and that science "is regarded as the quintessentially masculine intellectual activity." Internal medicine should take special note, since from the beginning it was "the link between clinical medicine and laboratory investigation [that] gave internal medicine a knowledge base competitive with surgical empiricism" (2).

The banking metaphor highlights the authors' concern that faculty who operate in the banking mode share only the end-product of their learning and discovery rather than the struggles of learning and the gratifications of discovery themselves. Stated differently, the metaphor says that banking faculty hand down their knowledge from on high, in sibylline fashion as it were, thereby distancing learners from the frustrating but ultimately crucial process of raising their own intellectual children.

The authors then shift the metaphor to a deeper and more elemental level. In some of their more striking language, they suggest that "banking education anesthetizes." In their view, banking education may even be like anesthesia during childbirth, which renders the woman a passive spectator; the physician now "usurps the woman's natural role during childbirth as *he* now 'gives birth' to the baby" (1, p 217; emphasis in the original). This echoes the Oxford English Dictionary, which notes that the roots of the word "educare," to raise children, lie deeper in the two Latin words "e ducere," to bring forth, which is, after all, what midwifery is all about.

In sum, midwife teachers, then, do the opposite of what banking teachers do. "Midwife teachers do not administer anesthesia" (1, p 217). They help learners to bring forth their fragile newborn thoughts; they assist in the emergence of consciousness; they encourage students to speak in their own voices. They say to students things like "What you're thinking is fine, but think more." They are willing to say "I don't know, but together we can figure this out." Problem-based learning, now becoming established in a wide variety of medical schools, thus may be said to represent a move away from banking and toward midwife education.

The metaphors are powerful and useful as far as they go, but like all metaphors, they weaken on closer scrutiny. Banking is not necessarily all bad; banks do serve their useful purposes. Some may not like the principle of usury (it is not permitted under Islam, for example), but we would probably miss banks if they disappeared. Money deposited in the bank does tend to be kept in a safe and an orderly way, and like knowledge deposited in learners' minds, money in the bank does acquire interest (in two senses: It grows, and it appeals).

What's more, the learning of certain skills calls for banking education as much as it does for midwife education. Do fragile newborn thoughts or personal voices need to be nurtured in learning to fly a jet plane—or to do a lumbar puncture? Learning tasks like these does have aspects—anxiety, confusion, and misperceptions, for example—that need to be brought forth, examined, and dealt with. But banking seems better than midwifery as the way to achieve clear, complete, unambiguous, and efficient transfer of task-related knowledge and experience. Now some would argue that "education" like this is not education at all, but "training." Our faithful Oxford English Dictionary informs us that the root of "training" is the French word "traine," to drag or to draw, with connotations of a forced process; the terms used to define the verb "to train," that is, "to subject to discipline" or "to condition," have a distinctly military ring. From the etymological point of view, therefore, training and education have relatively little in common. And from these reflections, it appears that the appropriate place for banking is in the realm of training, while education calls for more of the midwife. Medicine, being a rich and complex blend of the theoretical and the applied, calls for a mixture of training and education, in a proportion that depends on the particular aspect that's being learned.

While midwives play important roles in the birthing of babies, a great many babies have been born without the help of midwives or anyone else. What do midwives actually do? They coach, they encourage, they reassure, they look for trouble, they provide physical assistance, they provide experience; they've been there before. But in the final analysis, it is the mother who does most of the work, even when a midwife assists. By analogy, some would insist that while teachers may put everything they have into teaching, the hard labor of learning is ultimately done by the students themselves.

The concept of education as a bringing forth or raising up, whether by the students themselves or by students with their teachers, of course is not new. About 2,500 years ago, Socrates (3),

> pretending to complete ignorance , , , . queried all and sundry concerning those traditional virtues about which for one reason or another they might be expected to know and which, indeed they prided themselves on knowing.

The power of the Socratic method is inherent whether learning is a dialogue of two people or of a mind with itself. As a person teaches herself, she "elicits ideas from herself" by questioning, and tests those ideas by questioning herself again; she does with herself what Socrates did with other people (3, p xxvi). Self-assessment techniques, used increasingly in medicine, are thus in the grand tradition of Socratic teaching. (See Chapter 11, Mirror, Mirror.) "Women's Ways of Knowing" reminds us that teachers and learners share with each other the reflection and the refinement, the bringing forth and the raising up, when the education they are engaged in is authentic education.

REFERENCES

1. **Belenky MF, Clinchy BM, Goldberger NR, Tarule J.** Women's Ways of Knowing. The Development of Self, Voice and Mind. New York: Basic Books; 1986.
2. **Stevens R.** The curious career of internal medicine: functional ambivalence, social success. In: Maulitz RC, Long DE, Wood FC, eds. Grand Rounds: One Hundred Years of Internal Medicine. Philadelphia: University of Pennsylvania Press; 1988:343.
3. **Edman I, ed.** The Works of Plato. New York: Random House; 1928.

CHAPTER 22

Confidence Testing

How To Answer a Meta-Question

He who knows and knows that he knows is conceited; avoid him.
He who knows not and knows not that he knows not is a fool; instruct him.
He who knows and knows not that he knows is asleep; awaken him.
But he who knows not and knows that he knows not is a wise man;
    follow him.

ARAB PROVERB

*T*he venerable multiple choice question (MCQ) is firmly established as the principal tool for measuring the state of someone's medical knowledge, largely because our vast experience with MCQs gives them the unchallenged edge over other psychometric techniques. MCQs do their job so well that, in fact, the MCQ-based statistical perspective almost totally dominates our thinking about the evaluation of clinical competence. Even the most basic assumptions underlying their *modus operandi* are now accepted virtually without question.

Statistical thinking is, more generally, an instrument of great power. It is easy, therefore, to forget that the statistical "lens" introduces distortions into its picture of people's thinking. (Recall that statistics has been called "humanity with the tears wiped away.") As part of the statistical armamentarium, MCQs likewise filter medical reality, with results that are of particular concern, as follows. First, MCQs require examinees to categorize their answers as either "right" or "wrong." Much of medicine lends itself to this kind of black-and-white thinking, but much of it is incomplete, ambiguous, or conflicting. Not only does answering MCQs therefore fail to model faithfully most real clinical problem solving, but also it is difficult or even impossible to write MCQs for the many important but "fuzzy" clinical problems, that is, those that do not intrinsically lend themselves to the dichotomous categorization required by MCQs.

Secondly and more to the point, MCQs come up short at a deeper level: the all-or-none payoff associated with MCQs rewards guessing, which is why MCQs have acquired the sardonic alternative name of "multiple guess questions." But a reward system that encourages guessing is no laughing matter, principally since a system that rewards guessing rewards overconfidence, and overconfidence is not in the best interests of either physicians or patients.

Thirdly, a "right-wrong" scoring system assumes that the only knowledge worth anything (i.e., the only knowledge that is given credit) is *complete* knowledge. Incomplete or partial knowledge—knowledge that, while useful, isn't sufficiently clear or complete in people's minds for them to commit themselves unequivocally to a single answer—is considered worthless. Right-or-wrong scoring of MCQs thus penalizes any impulse to hedge, or worse, ignores and ultimately extinguishes hedging, even when hedging would more accurately reflect the state of a person's usable knowledge.

In its present form, therefore, MCQ testing throws away valuable information about a learner's state of mind. But in this instance the information being wasted is not only about factual *knowledge* per se, but also about *confidence* in that knowledge. Diamond and Forrester have clearly framed the fundamental distinction between the two (1). Knowledge, in their view, is the kind of response that is given to questions of fact, for example, "Does this patient have a peptic ulcer?" In contrast, confidence is the response to a question about a question, which the authors refer to as a "meta-question;" in this instance, the meta-question is "How sure are you of your answer to the question about whether the patient has an ulcer?"

Stated differently, it is the difference between a physician's assertion that "there's a 60 percent chance this treatment will work" (knowledge) versus the assertion that "there's a 10% chance I know what I'm talking about" (confidence). Recognition of the difference has profound implications for medicine, since the ability to adjust your level of confidence to match your knowledge is critical in coping with the inevitable uncertainty of medicine. (See Chapter 25, A Touch of Cancer.) Unfortunately, making this adjustment is difficult for most people, physicians included. Indeed, one thoughtful student of this problem has concluded that (2)

> Physicians . . . will acknowledge medicine's uncertainty once its presence is forced into conscious awareness, yet at the same time will continue to conduct their practices as if uncertainty did not exist.

It is important to point out that, while MCQs both reinforce overconfidence and, at the same time, fail altogether to assess or even recognize confidence, the broader discipline of statistics explicitly acknowledges both the difference between knowledge and confidence and the importance of that difference. It is, after all, biomedical statistics, that hardest and most quantitative of sciences, that uses the *confidence interval* as one of its most important quantitative measures (3). In using this term, statisticians are telling us clearly that the main purpose of their discipline—all their theory, their algebra, their hard numbers—is to adjust people's level of confidence in their (intrinsically uncertain) factual knowledge, rather than to influence the content of that knowledge per se.

While the dominance of "right-wrong" MCQs implies that confidence isn't worth measuring, can't be measured, or both, an important new discipline of confidence testing has emerged over the past 30 years, indicating that neither of these pessimistic conclusions is justified (4). The basic theory of *confidence testing* is simple but subtle. Instead of forcing you into making artificially confident "yes-or no" choices among answers, confidence testing allows you to express your degree of confidence ("shades of gray") in *all* the answers to a particular question, even though only one of those answers is actually correct. Thus, if you are reasonably, but not completely, sure answer A is right you might express your degree of confidence in that answer by assigning it a probability value of 0.7 (on a scale ranging from 0.0, which means you are certain an answer is *not* correct, to 1.0, which means you are certain it is). Now if you also think B might be correct but are less sure, you might assign it a value of 0.3, while C, which you are almost sure isn't correct, might get a 0.1. A state of complete uncertainty about any answer would be expressed by choosing 0.5 for all three options.

As a way of getting a handle on confidence, this straight probabilistic approach is a step in the right direction, but, as it happens, direct selection of probabilities is not an effective way to go about the task. The reason is quite simple: when people use probability values to express their preferences they soon learn that the payoff over many questions is greater if they place most or all of their confidence in one preferred answer, however limited their actual confidence in that answer might be. By so doing, they in effect recreate the present "right-wrong" MCQ scoring system. While this self-defeating property of probabilities appears to be a fairly intractable psychometric barrier, Brown and Shuford pointed out a way around it some years ago (5). Working, interestingly enough, in the area of government intelligence, they showed that when people are required to choose from a set of specially designed numerical payoffs (i.e., positive or negative score points) covering the entire range of confidence levels they will, over time, express their confidence more accurately than if they directly indicate their estimate of the probability that each answer is correct.

Thus, under this special reward (scoring) system, you gain moderately (i.e., you receive a moderate but not a very large number of points) when you indicate very high confidence in the correctness of answers that are, in fact, correct. As you indicate less and less confidence in what turn out to be correct answers, the payoff (number of points) drops gradually, reaching 0 points when you are completely uncertain; that is, the expression of true uncertainty (which in probability terms would be expressed as 0.5) is neither rewarded nor penalized. Your score then becomes rapidly negative (progressively more points are subtracted from your score) as you indicate stronger and stronger confidence that correct answers are wrong.

While these numerical scores make intuitive sense, they were not arrived at casually but were calculated from equations known technically as "reproducing scoring functions." Sometimes also referred to as "scoring functions that encourage honesty," the real punch of these scoring systems lies in the fact that they allow you to maximize your score if—and only if—the confidence you have in your knowledge is perfectly "calibrated" to the correctness of that knowledge. That is, your score will be highest in the long run if 50% of the answers are, in fact, correct in the group of answers for which you were willing to accept no score points, thereby expressing complete lack of confidence that the answer was either right or wrong (i.e., equivalent to a probability of correctness of 0.5); if 90% are correct in the group where you chose a number of points corresponding to the confidence level specifically equivalent to a probability of correctness of 0.9; if only 10% of answers are correct in the group where you were willing to risk the negative points corresponding to the low confidence level specifically equivalent to a probability of correctness of only 0.1; and so on for groups of answers assigned over the entire range of confidence levels.

This form of confidence testing can be implemented using pencil and paper (for MCQs with up to three answers, one of which is correct). Using this approach, it is possible to tell the degree to which lack of knowledge versus inappropriate confidence accounts for less than optimal test scores (4). Importantly, the statistical reliability for the knowledge component of test scores increases when scores are corrected for inappropriate confidence. It is also possible using extensions of this technique to assess whether a test taker is overconfident or underconfident, and by how much. For example, someone is said to be overconfident if only 20% of their answers are correct among all those assigned the number of points that expresses a confidence equal to, say, a 0.9 probability of their being right. An underconfident person is the opposite, that is, one whose answers are correct 70% of the time in the group assigned points expressing confidence equal to a low probability of their being right, for example, 0.3. Interestingly enough, when confidence was measured this way, even second-year medical students were found to overvalue substantially the correctness of their answers, which perhaps isn't surprising in view of their extensive prior experience with "right-wrong" MCQs. Even more interestingly, exposure to confidence testing helped students learn not to overvalue the correctness of their knowledge or, stated differently, their confidence became better "calibrated" to the actual state of their knowledge (4).

Any way you measure it, confidence that is miscalibrated, either too high or too low, may be at least as much a problem in clinical medicine as *lack* of knowledge per se. The effects of inappropriate lack of confidence may be less obvious than those of overconfidence, although underconfidence can be a serious stumbling block for physicians in its own right, contributing to excessive testing and use of consultants or, at the extreme, the inability to make decisions at all. In general, however, physicians are extremely wary of underconfidence, their concern being that underconfidence, or even the appearance of it, undermines patient trust, and that lack of patient trust fundamentally compromises their ability to treat. Unfortunately, overconfidence causes physicians to jump to inappropriate diagnostic and therapeutic conclusions, fail to learn when they need to learn, and lose patients' trust when their confidence is found to have been misplaced (2). (See Chapter 5, The Voytovich Solution and Chapter 25, A Touch of Cancer.)

If, in fact, it is "the 'vital office' of scientific medicine to develop systems of thought and action that will permit physicians to account more fully for both the certainties and uncertainties that shape their practices" (2), then scientific medicine needs to reconsider the unspoken effects of the "right-wrong mentality" on our ability to deal with those certainties and uncertainties. In particular, it needs to rethink the current, almost exclusive reliance on multiple-choice questions and the contribution of that evaluation format to miscalibration of physician confidence. In this regard, effective techniques for recognizing, assessing, and calibrating physician confidence, such as the technique of confidence testing or similar measures, are among the most important "systems of thought and action" we can develop for carrying out this vital office.

REFERENCES

1. **Diamond GA, Forrester JS.** Metadiagnosis. An epistemologic model of clinical judgment. Am J Med. 1983;75:129-37.
2. **Katz J.** Acknowledging uncertainty: the confrontation of knowledge and ignorance. In: The Silent World of Doctor and Patient. New York: Free Press; 1984:165-206.
3. **Gardner MJ, Altman DG, eds.** Statistics with Confidence. Confidence Intervals and Statistical Guidelines. London: BMJ Publishing Co.; 1989.
4. **Rippey RM, Voytovich AE.** Linking knowledge, realism and diagnostic reasoning by computer-assisted confidence testing. Journal of Computer Based Instruction. 1983;9:88-97.
5. **Brown TA, Shuford EH.** Quantifying uncertainty into numerical probabilities for the reporting of intelligence. ARPA Report R-1185-ARPA. Santa Monica, CA: Rand; 1973.

CHAPTER *23*

The Technologies of Education

~

Sizzle and Steak

*A*n experienced observer has commented that you can tell when an academic internist is giving a lecture because the opening words are always "First slide, please." This sardonic vignette underscores the degree to which slide projectors are now taken for granted; part of the educational landscape that goes almost unnoticed—except when the bulb burns out. Yet not so long ago the "magic lantern" was a technological wonder.

No sooner had slide projectors lost their magic, however, when reel-to-reel tape recorders appeared on the scene, then it was audiocassettes, followed, of course, by computers, and the promise of high-tech teaching and learning seemed to explode all over the place. The list of educationally relevant technological wonders is long and grows almost daily: electronic networks, electronic literature searching, videotaped information and instruction, CDs containing whole libraries of text and images, computer-assisted instruction (CAI) packages, computer-based exams (CBX), keypad feedback (electronic response systems that instantly and anonymously survey an audience, tally the results, and display them on a screen), palmtops, and now compu-television. Information technology increasingly absorbs medical educators' energy, attention, enthusiasm—and funds.

And why shouldn't it? Today, everything from the basic structure of matter to the behavior of their "chaotic" macrosystems is being rethought in terms of information, so it seems only natural that medical

123

teaching, learning, and understanding, which are so information-intensive, should stand to be revolutionized by these powerful new systems. A basic dictum in marketing is "Sell the sizzle, not the steak." Curiously, despite all the "sizzle"—that is, the promise and the excitement—hard evidence for the existence of educational "steak"—substantial, measurable improvement in learning and medical practice as a product of these technologies—is minimal, at best. Why?

To begin with, educational success is a moving target. The surface attractiveness of a new educational system, the enthusiasm and loyalty it engenders, and the apparent obviousness of its advantages, any of which might once have sufficed for it to flourish, are no longer quite enough. The psychometricians are just waiting out there to see whether we are justified in claiming that the latest in educational wonders really "works," and their measurements are now sensitive to both medical knowledge and clinical skills. (See Chapter 26, What Can Doctors Do?) Clinicians themselves are increasingly professional skeptics (1), given a history strewn with the wreckage of tests and treatments that initially seemed obviously better but were later abandoned because they were shown to be ineffective, toxic, or both. As a consequence, medical education itself is increasingly held to more rigorous standards than it once was; we have entered what might be called the era of evidence-based education.

For example, as recently as the late 1980s, the CBX was seen as having obvious advantages for testing both knowledge and skills. Its use as part of so-called "high stakes" medical examinations seemed inevitable, so much so that enormous investments were made in computerized equipment and testing facilities. But as of the mid-1990s, CBX is still not a part of those exams. What happened? Hard evidence, obtained with considerable difficulty and at considerable cost, revealed that CBX is indeed an effective way of testing knowledge. But the investigators didn't stop there; they asked the right follow-up question: Is CBX *better* at testing knowledge than more conventional, and cheaper, paper-and-pencil tests? That is, is it more efficient or reliable or valid? And does it tap into anything beyond knowledge, a previously unmeasured clinical "something extra" that contributes to high-quality medical care? The answer was no to all of the above; indeed, in some respects, CBX was actually less accurate and reliable than traditional testing modes. Given the large amounts of money and effort that had been sunk into its development, not to mention its undeniable "Star Trek" allure, the difficult, evidence-based decision to hold off on including CBX as part of a national licensing examination was a courageous one.

There is, moreover, increasing recognition that Lewis Thomas was right when, reflecting on the use of technology in medicine generally, he suggested that much of what initially appears to be "high technology" turns out instead to be "halfway technology" (2). The iron lung (the Drinker respirator), widely used in the treatment of bulbar paralytic polio, is a prime example of halfway technology: a dramatic, sometimes life-saving and seemingly high-tech device that, at least in retrospect, is seen to be clumsy, nonspecific, and inefficient, and that gets at the problem when most of the damage is already done.

In Thomas's view, the use of a halfway technology such as the iron lung is a sign that knowledge about a problem is seriously deficient. The Salk vaccine, in contrast, is a true high technology: it depends on a deep understanding of the nature of the problem, and it is elegant, highly specific, inexpensive, and gets at the problem before it starts (primary prevention). (See Chapter 38, Education, Patients, and the Public.) Seen in this light, CAI, video-based learning, keypad feedback systems, and the like, despite their outward glamour and seemingly endless promise, are more halfway than true high technologies.

The major problem in the realm of undergraduate medical education, for example, appears to be the traditional paradigm of high faculty-controlled teaching plus passive, memorization-based learning itself, rather than lack of powerful electronic information systems. And active, learner-centered, problem-solving learning is emerging in this situation as a high technology, a kind of educational Salk vaccine, if you will. Further underscoring the point, inexpensive hand-held cards, color-coded on one side, have been shown to do just about everything for group learning that an expensive electronic audience response system can do.

This said, it is important to distinguish these views from a Luddite (anti-technology) position, and to point out in fairness the small amount of hard evidence that has emerged, slowly and painfully, demonstrating certain advantages of new information technologies over traditional education methods (3). Moreover, electronic mail and electronic literature searching, for example—unsexy, plain vanilla, relatively mature technologies—have helped educators implement effective problem-based learning. And videotaping has clearly opened up a whole new dimension of teaching and learning in interpersonal medical work, including interviewing, counseling, and the like.

Unfortunately, even a demonstration that a new information technology is more effective than medical education in the old ways doesn't get at the critical underlying question of specificity. Ever since the infamous so-called "Dr. Fox" experiments, which were designed to distinguish the educational impact of style from that of substance (sizzle vs. steak), it has been clear just how powerful nonspecific, noncognitive factors can be in learning. A factor such as "expressiveness" (attractive presentation and personal style, with its associated activation of learners' attentiveness, interest, and sense of mastery) can be demonstrably a good thing (i.e., increased learning) or a bad one (i.e., distorted perceptions of what and how much was learned) (4,5). Oliver Sacks's vignette of the group of aphasic patients fully engaged with the image of the President on television despite not being able to understand a single word of his speech is a poignant affirmation of the phenomenon (6).

Certainly, the excitement, enthusiasm, and anxiety generated by the new information technologies suggest that Dr. Fox himself is busily at work here. But only time, plus a great deal of hard work and a properly skeptical mind set, will tell whether new information technologies actually improve education in meaningful ways, and if so, how. Traps for the unwary abound. One important concern is the difficulty of keeping technical advances separate from improvements in the richness, structure, and uses of knowledge. Using MEDLINE to search the literature electronically, for example, allows you to comb through six or seven million published papers in a twinkling but, by itself, does not improve either the quality of what you find or your ability to interpret it. (See Chapter 3, Music Lessons.) Even within the narrow realm of technology, it is easy to mistake promise for reality. For example, electronic bulletin boards and electronic mail are widely regarded as labor-saving, productivity-enhancing technologies, yet when you take into account the difficulties of acquiring equipment, learning arcane and rapidly changing commands, waiting for systems that are down, and wading through the drifts of unwanted or useless information, it's apparent these systems may not save labor or time at all, and may even, on balance, be detrimental (7).

The promise of the new information technologies will probably be realized only when we acquire deep understanding in two complementary areas. First, we need to know much more about the noncognitive side of learning. How does expressiveness really work? What can and can't it do? Where can it go wrong? How can it be used most effectively? And second, we need to develop a new and substantially more sophisticated understanding of the structure of information and the representation of meaning. The recent development of a system for classifying, identifying, and marking the context of sentences in the medical literature is an example of such an advance (8). Without such progress we are likely to have to live indefinitely with halfway information technologies in education; with it, teaching and learning could be enormously enhanced.

REFERENCES

1. Evidence-Based Medicine Working Group. Evidence-based medicine. A new approach to teaching the practice of medicine. JAMA. 1992;268:2420-5.
2. Thomas L. The technology of medicine. In: The Lives of a Cell. Notes of a Biology Watcher. New York: Viking Press; 1974:31-6.
3. Cohen PA, Dacanay LS. Computer-based instruction and health professions education: a meta-analysis of outcomes. Education and the Health Professions. 1992;15:259-81.
4. Ware JE Jr, Williams RG. The Dr. Fox effect: a study of lecturer effectiveness and ratings of instruction. J Med Educ. 1975;50:149-56.
5. Williams RG, Ware JE Jr. An extended visit with Dr. Fox: validity of student satisfaction with instruction rations after repeated exposures to a lecturer. Am Educ Res J. 1977;14:449-57.
6. Sacks O. The President's Speech. In: The Man Who Mistook His Wife for a Hat. New York: Summit Books; 1985:76-80.
7. Stoll C. Silicon Snake Oil. Second Thoughts on the Information Highway. New York: Doubleday, 1995.
8. Purcell GP, Shortliffe EH. Contextual models of clinical publications for enhancing retrieval from full-text databases. Nineteenth Annual Symposium on Computer Applications in Medical Care; October 28–November 1, 1995; New Orleans: McGraw-Hill; 1995:851-7.

CHAPTER 24

The Right Hand of Claude

Reflections on Becoming an Expert

A t the hospital in Boston where I did my residency, surgical residents in the later years of their training could elect a two-month rotation on the service of a distinguished general surgeon—Claude Welch, if I remember right. I once asked someone who had been through the rotation what residents actually did while on that service; he said, "During the first month we watched what Welch did with his right hand; during the second month we watched what he did with his left."

In thinking about the more general problem of how people learn to become truly expert, I've been increasingly impressed with the deeper educational implications of that resident's account. Basically, he was saying, "Even for someone who is already quite skillful, an important first step in moving to higher levels of mastery is first to break a complex skill down into its component parts. Only after you've mastered the parts separately can you put them together into the finished performance."

Serious students of the problem have described a similar but more general model for acquiring expertise, based largely on observations in other fields (1). It begins at the most basic level with the acquisition of "skills-based" performance—patterns of thought and action governed by stored patterns of "pre-programmed" instructions, which the mavens refer to as "schemata." These schemata are reminiscent of what my surgical colleague absorbed by watching Claude Welch's right hand. As experience increases, the process metamorphoses into "rules-based" performance in which solutions to familiar problems are governed by stored rules of the "if X, then Y" variety.

As people become experts, the process ultimately reaches a "knowledge-based" level of performance, one that depends on synthetic thought (that is, requiring conscious analysis and stored knowledge) in dealing with new situations. Paradoxically, novices are forced to figure everything out from first principles, which they obviously can't do very well until they have acquired the requisite "schemata." Experts, in contrast, seldom have to resort to such knowledge-based functioning since they have "a much larger repertoire of schemata and problem-solving rules than novices, and they are formulated at a more abstract level" (2). At the same time, the mark of an expert is the ability to use knowledge-based reasoning, when it is needed, very efficiently indeed (2). (See Chapter 4, Is Basic Science Necessary?)

The training of experts in most fields, including medicine, is a high-intensity enterprise. That is to say, a great deal of learning is compressed into every day of training (and many nights as well), leaving little time or energy for anything else. This routine often continues without respite for years. As the author and commentator Alistair Cooke once remarked, all you need to do to become an expert is, in effect, get up every day and devote yourself entirely to the task at hand, over and over, until the day comes when you wake up and find yourself one of the competent ones of your generation.

Training this intense raises legitimate concerns about dehumanization and exploitation of students, but the intensity itself seems somehow connected with the idea of reaching beyond ordinary levels of achievement. It is as though experts know that students must reach a kind of "critical mass" of skill—the once-you've-learned-it-you-never-forget-it level, as when you learn to ride a bicycle—before they can cross over into the forbidden territory of high-level mastery. Creating this much-prized "critical mass" may simply require a certain level of pressure; a too leisurely pace or a too casual attitude may simply allow students to slip back too much every day, may not permit them to regain every day what they've lost from the day before, then move ahead to reach the necessary "fusion threshold." Intensity may also operate at an attitudinal level, conveying a meta-message about the extreme importance of what students are learning.

High-level training is associated with low student–faculty ratios, tailored programs, private lessons. But while a few learners become experts entirely without being part of a group, even the surgical residents who spent two months alone with Claude Welch were very much connected to their peers the rest of the time, as are most students on the way to high-level mastery in medicine or other disciplines.

As members of a group, those who are becoming experts share not only in the satisfactions of learning but also in the disappointments and the setbacks, the gripes and the black humor, supporting each other through the training process in all its intensity. Peers teach each other, particularly in medicine (3), and peers supply much of the excitement and enthusiasm needed to stay the course. Peer pressure also contributes a good measure of the competition, the discipline, and the values attached to expert training, as well as the benchmarks against which students measure their progress (4). It is surely not an accident, then, that becoming an expert is usually at least as much a social as an individual matter.

The teachers of expert-level performance also must have a unique blend of abilities: the ability to perform at a high level *and* the ability to reflect on performance, both in themselves and in their students (5). Great performers may or may not have the ability to reflect, which probably explains why not all great performers are great teachers. Many images are associated with the master teacher—*professor, scholar, mentor, guru*—and many of these images make sense for disciplines that primarily involve abstract, intellectual work. For the performing professions, however—music and theater, design and dance, architecture, law, medicine—where the ability to act is as important as the ability to think, coach is probably the term that best fits the reality of the master teacher. And while coaching in the professions has begun to receive serious attention (5), the theory and practice of coaching still need a great deal of work, particularly in medicine.

The concept of coaching resonates with the four-component cycle of experiential learning described by Lewin, Dewey, Piaget, and others. Kolb's synthesis of these components suggests that students learning in the "experiential" mode must be given the opportunity to participate fully in all four linked aspects of the cycle, that is, to

- Involve themselves fully, openly, and without bias in new experiences;

- Observe and reflect on their experiences from many perspectives, which allows them to formulate the nature of the problems they've been dealing with;

- Explore and create concepts that allow them to integrate the problems they have faced into critically appraised patterns, principles, theories; and

- Use these patterns, principles, and theories to make decisions and solve the next set of unfamiliar problems (6).

Coaching medical residents, then, means providing them with experience in managing a good mix of familiar and unknown problems. It involves leading them back and forth between experiences and reflection on those experiences through reading, discussion (particularly Socratic), feedback, modeling, introspection, and input from a variety of disciplines. It involves helping students learn to apply "standardizing" techniques (2), that is, principles, tips, and rules, such as learning to make complete and precise problem lists, to use flow sheets, algorithms, heuristics (rules of thumb), and the like (7). (See Chapter 5, The Voytovich Solution, and Chapter 25, A Touch of Cancer.) Lastly, it involves moving students along the path of graduated, increasingly independent decision making and responsibility.

Even the best coaching won't be effective, however, unless it happens in a setting that contains many other important features of an environment that supports learning. At the level of residency training in internal medicine, many (but not all) of these features are captured in the so-called "Special Requirements" developed by the Residency Review Committee in Internal Medicine, the criteria on which residency training programs are based and on which their quality is judged. This clinical learning environment includes obvious physical elements such as hospital versus outpatient or home care settings, but others less obvious may be just as important. Examples include the bedside as a place for teaching in addition to the conference room, an abundance of well-organized and easily accessible information resources, and a setting that is a realistic reflection of practice. And then there are organizational features of the teaching environment, including

- **Balance** between redundancy and variation of experience—enough repetition to reinforce learning, enough diversity to stimulate, to teach the fine points.

- **Pacing** that slows things down when residents are learning complex skills, allowing them to "concentrate on what the right hand is doing," and that speeds things up when they are learning how to do things that need to be done under pressure.

- **A safe climate** that allows residents to experiment, to learn hard lessons from their inevitable mistakes without feeling they are bad people (4). This is critical, since one feature of expertise is making the fewest possible mistakes, and continuously learning from those mistakes (2).

• **A peer group** that generally pulls together.

As Kolb points out, a certain degree of tension is intrinsic to the job of coaching since, on the one hand, experiential learning, particularly at the expert level, requires learners to act and reflect at the same time, but, on the other hand, it is difficult to be concrete and also be "theoretical" at the same time (6). The pedagogical challenge to coaching is correspondingly great, therefore, since it requires coaches to support the simultaneous exercise of abilities that are polar opposites. Claude Welch, it seems, was a master teacher precisely because he knew how to help his residents move back and forth between being actors and observers, between immediate, concrete work as his OR team assistants and analytic detachment as active, experiential learners.

All learning, but particularly "real world" (rather than simulated) experiential learning, also requires learners to continually push the envelope, to move repeatedly out of the comfort zone of knowledge and skills already mastered. The philosopher Hegel said on this point that "any experience that does not violate expectation is not worthy of the name experience." If, however, learners get pushed too far, they will be "left paralyzed by insecurity, incapable of ineffective action" (6). Effective learning therefore requires learners to encounter many things that rip the fabric of experience, but these rips then need somehow to be "magically" repaired, so that the learner can face the next day, a bit changed, but still the same person (6).

Looking at all this complexity, it's a wonder anyone ever learns to be an expert, but of course people do, every day of the week. At the same time, it couldn't hurt if we got to be more expert on how to make that happen.

REFERENCES

1. **Rasmussen J, Jensen A.** Mental procedures in real-life tasks: a case study of electronic trouble-shooting. Ergonomics. 1974;17:293-307.
2. **Leape LL.** Error in medicine. JAMA. 1994;272:1851-7.
3. **Mizrahi T.** Getting Rid of Patients. Contradictions in the Socialization of Physicians. New Brunswick, NJ: Rutgers University Press; 1986.
4. **Bosk C.** Forgive and Remember. Managing Medical Failure. Chicago: University of Chicago Press; 1979.
5. **Schön DA.** Educating the Reflective Practitioner: Toward a New

Design for Teaching and Learning in the Professions. San Francisco: Jossey-Bass; 1988.

6. **Kolb DA.** Experiential Learning. Experience as the Source of Learning and Development. Englewood Cliffs, NJ: PTR Prentice Hall; 1984.

7. **McDonald CJ.** Medical heuristics. The silent adjudicators of clinical practice. Ann Intern Med. 1996;124:56-62.

CHAPTER 25

A Touch of Cancer

Teaching about Uncertainty

*T*olerance for uncertainty is a characteristic that particularly distinguishes medical generalists. But all of medicine is shot through
with uncertainty, and everyone who practices medicine, generalist and
specialist alike, needs to become skilled in dealing with it.

Teaching about medical uncertainty—what it is, how to recognize it,
measure it, manage it, work with it—is thus a fundamental task for
medical education. Throughout the history of medicine, tolerance for
and skill in dealing with uncertainty have been seen as things you either
bring with you into medicine or you don't. But in the past 100 years or
so, a science of uncertainty has quietly been developing—in mathematics, physics, economics—and, fortunately, more recently within medicine as well, providing a new kind of leverage for improving everyone's
ability to work under uncertainty conditions. The pace of development
in the field has accelerated markedly in recent years, with implications
for medicine and medical teaching that are just now beginning to be
recognized.

The common denominator of the various approaches to uncertainty is the assumption that complex, seemingly random events are determined by discrete, definable, quantifiable factors, and, moreover, that
these factors can be captured as symbols and manipulated according to
the principles of mathematical logic. Of course, epidemiologists began
mathematical modeling of uncertainty in their own particular universe
decades ago. But the epidemiologists counted, measured, predicted in

a universe that, by definition, consisted of populations, not individual patients. The conceptual breakthrough that led to the first application of quantitative thinking to the uncertainties surrounding individual patients is popularly ascribed to a radiologist, Lee Lusted (1). Thus were born the disciplines of clinical epidemiology and its cousin, medical decision analysis, examples, perhaps, of a true scientific revolution in medicine (2) that is less than 30 years old. The development of clinical epidemiology and decision analysis in the intervening years has been vigorous, with the proliferation of research (3) and the publication of several important textbooks (references 4 and 5, for example).

At the core of these complex and diverse fields lies the "probabilistic" concept of predictive value. Predictive value is a mathematical variant of Bayes' theorem, a concept that originated with an obscure British cleric in the mid-eighteenth century and that has come to dominate mathematical statistics in the past half-century (6). In simplest terms, the idea of predictive value tells us that, while at any given moment the state of our knowledge about a clinical situation is uncertain (a question whether or not a patient has cancer, for example), our initial degree of uncertainty can be specified in terms of a probability, or likelihood. Every new piece of clinical data we obtain then has the potential for modifying ideally, lessening—that uncertainty. Indeed, the task of clinical medicine can be viewed as essentially a continuing, iterative process in which we use items of clinical information to convert pre-existing likelihoods (prior probabilities) into new ones (posterior probabilities or predictive values). Use of the term *predictive value* refers to an assumption that the new (presumably greater) level of assurance resulting from new information predicts the patient's true medical condition more accurately than the previous level (7).

A particularly crucial, yet not intuitively obvious property of predictive values is that an item of medical information has greater or lesser impact on the likelihood of a diagnosis depending on how high or low the probability is to start with. In a situation of low disease prevalence, for example (testing an asymptomatic person off the street for multiple sclerosis), a positive result from even a reasonably sensitive and specific test does not make that disease much more likely. In contrast, a positive result from that very same test applied in a high prevalence situation (a patient referred to a multiple sclerosis clinic because of blurred vision in one eye) may essentially establish a diagnosis. More generally, an identical test applied at low, medium, and high prevalences can be said to operate in three very different ways, that is, screening, diagnostic, and confirmatory modes, respectively.

The implications of using probabilistic methods for understanding and managing uncertainty are in principle tremendous, for both outcomes and costs, and for both clinicians and patients. But despite the efforts of many to draw probabilistic reasoning into the clinical mainstream (8,9), clinicians still generally find it very difficult to use explicit, quantitative probabilistic reasoning at the bedside. And despite at least one randomized, controlled prospective educational intervention trial demonstrating that a probabilistic curriculum actually changes physicians' test-ordering behavior (10), the response of most medical faculty to the idea of teaching probabilistic reasoning has been underwhelming.

Physicians almost certainly use estimates of uncertainty and probability all the time in implicit, intuitive ways, but explicit, quantitative probabilistic reasoning is complex and unfamiliar, even counterintuitive, to most physicians and medical faculty (11). It isn't exactly surprising, therefore, that probabilistic reasoning has diffused so slowly into the practicing and teaching communities. But probabilistic reasoning may be up against other, deeper difficulties as well.

To begin with, all probabilistic reasoning rests on the fundamental assumption of absolute (crisp) distinctions between states, for example, disease versus nondisease, cure versus noncure. Now, while probabilistic reasoning can assess the likelihood of being one or another crisply defined state, it is best at doing so when dealing with single items of information, particularly when that information itself is precise, that is, numbers. For the most part, however, clinicians can't limit themselves to single items of information; indeed, they deal all the time with hundreds or thousands of chunks of information, washing over them in waves. And most clinical information is captured and expressed in the subtle and ambiguous medium of words (along with some images), rather than in numbers.

To claim that it can manage medical uncertainty, therefore, any robust system will at least need to be able to handle the "surface" issue of patients' membership in crisply defined states as they are expressed in the everyday welter of words, sights, sounds, smells, and tactile sensations. But there's a second problem, deeper and more subtle than the first: patients can simultaneously occupy several different, nonmutually exclusive, ambiguously defined medical states. Unfortunately, there's a little problem here: the concept of ambiguously defined states simply challenges virtually all of Western logical thought, which, from Aristotle on, has been based on the use of absolute or crisp definitions.

Now, it just so happens that over the last 30 years, a new branch of mathematical logic has developed that does not assume crisp definition of states (6). Known by the inexact and somewhat misleading term *fuzzy logic*, this field has advanced rapidly and has had a substantial effect on mathematical theory and engineering practice, although its impact on medicine has so far been limited.

The fundamental tenets of fuzzy logic may be made clearer by recalling the old sardonic allusion to someone being "just a little bit pregnant." Now everyone *knows*, of course, that pregnancy is, first, a crisply defined state, a "pure case" if there ever was one. This crisp definition is an essential prerequisite for a second universal assumption about pregnancy, namely that membership in the pregnant state is *exclusive*, that is, incompatible with membership in the state of nonpregnancy, and vice versa. And clearly you can only be exclusively in one state or another if the boundary between them is sharp. The irony of "a little bit pregnant" therefore comes from the inference that someone can simultaneously be *both* partly pregnant and partly nonpregnant, which, in light of the common wisdom about the nature of the pregnant state, is absurd.

But think, now, about the clinical realities: Is an ectopic pregnancy really a pregnancy? And to exactly what extent is a woman pregnant if her intrauterine fetus is seriously malformed and aborts spontaneously? And how should we view the pregnancy that is unwanted and rejected by the parents? The simple reality is that the real world simply does not always respect crisp definitions or accommodate exclusive membership in specific states, even when it comes to motherhood. Or, looked at from a different angle, a woman can be simultaneously pregnant and nonpregnant, but only if each of the boundaries of the two states is blurred or "fuzzy," which, in turn, allows membership in a state to become nonexclusive. No wonder Bayesian reasoning has run into trouble in medicine!

Pregnancy is one of the more obvious examples of crisp distinction that doesn't square with the real world, but it certainly isn't the only one. In fact, partial inclusion in several ambiguously defined states is commonplace in medicine. Think about the many abnormal tissues classified as cancer on morphological grounds—thyroid, prostate, desmoid—that neither invade nor kill. Are they really malignant? Or, conversely, think about tumors called histologically benign that prove lethal because they occur in critical locations. Consider two average physicians, otherwise comparable in every respect, one of whom is not board-certified because he scored a single point lower than his neighbor, who receives all the privileges of certification. Think of terminally ill patients denied certain interventions that will relieve intractable suffering because any intervention that will hasten a patient's demise is exclusively assigned to the crisp category of "physician-assisted suicide" rather than the fuzzier category of "allowing patients to die."

The drive toward exclusive classifications in crisply defined states is powerful, fueled not only by 2,000 years of Aristotelian cultural tradition but also by the compelling personal as well as social need for clarity, certainty, and authority on the part of patients, physicians, insurance companies, epidemiologists—in fact, by nearly everyone who deals with clinical medicine. And, indeed, the fuzzy concept of partial membership in multiple, ambiguously defined states is tricky, something that can easily slide into sloppy thinking and distort reality. The idea that someone has "a touch of cancer" is not yet easy to live with.

At the end of the day, however, we have little choice but to come to grips with uncertainty, whether as probability or ambiguity. And although we've just begun to appreciate both the challenges and opportunities of the undertaking, we can be pleased that medicine and medical teaching have headed bravely out into this world, the little-known territory of prior and posterior likelihoods and ambiguous fuzzy states. That's the world of our patients and their problems.

REFERENCES

1. **Lusted LB.** Introduction to Medical Decision Making. Springfield, IL: Thomas; 1968.
2. **Kuhn TS.** The Structure of Scientific Revolutions. 2nd ed. Chicago: University of Chicago Press; 1970.
3. **Kahneman D, Slovic P, Tversky A, eds.** Judgment Under Uncertainty: Heuristics and Biases. New York: Cambridge University Press; 1982.
4. **Sackett DL, Haynes R, Guyatt GH, Tugwell P.** Clinical Epidemiology. A Basic Science for Clinical Medicine. 2nd ed. Boston: Little, Brown; 1991.
5. **Weinstein MC, Fineberg HV.** Clinical Decision Analysis. Philadelphia: WB Saunders; 1980.
6. **McNeil D, Freiberger P.** Fuzzy Logic. The Revolutionary Computer Technology that is Changing Our World. New York: Touchstone; 1993.
7. **Davidoff F.** Clinical medicine as a hard science. Clin Invest Med. 1981;4:57-81.

8. **Sox HC Jr, Blatt MA, Higgins MC, Marton KI.** Medical Decision Making. Boston: Butterworths; 1988.
9. **Bursztajn H, Feinbloom RI, Hamm RM, Brodsky A.** Medical Choices, Medical Chances. How Patients, Families and Physicians Can Cope with Uncertainty. New York: Delacorte Press; 1981.
10. **Davidoff F, Goodspeed R, Clive J.** Changing test ordering behavior. A randomized controlled trial comparing probabilistic reasoning with cost-containment education. Med Care. 1989; 27:45-58.
11. **Berwick D, Feinberg HV, Weinstein MC.** When doctors meet numbers. Am J Med. 1981;71:991-8.

CHAPTER 26

What Can Doctors Do?

Assessing Clinical Skills

All professions, medicine included, can be thought of and learned at four separate but interconnected levels: knowledge (what you know), skills or competence (what you can do), performance (what you actually do), and outcome (what the results are).

Learning at each level (optimally) includes an assessment (measurement, evaluation) component. Unfortunately, most learners see assessment as being, at best, less central than other more obvious, even glamorous, parts of learning or, at worst, a burden and a threat. But like it or not, assessment lies at the heart of the process, a critical link in the continuous learning feedback loop. (See Chapter 11, Mirror, Mirror.) Learning without assessment is therefore like sailing in the fog: You can do it, but it's hard to get where you're going without running on the rocks. Assessment is like radar: it won't navigate for you, but it shows you where things are, tells you if you're making progress and if you're in the right direction. Indeed, many knowledgeable people ascribe the recent disastrous failures of medical education in various countries around the world largely to a lack of standardized national examinations and other evaluation systems, with the resultant lack of overall medical education quality control.

Some even argue that evaluation is "The Force," the unappreciated silent partner that actually drives education. In the United States, this view is particularly prevalent when it comes to national licensing and certifying examinations, which are seen as determining what students, residents, and faculty consider important, and hence what learners learn and how they learn it. As reflected in the recent Robert Wood Johnson Foundation report, "Medical education in transition," however, the force of national standard-setting examinations is not universally seen as benign (1). According to this view, such examinations may not, in fact, reflect the knowledge that students really need in order to practice the best medicine; they may stifle exploration and creativity; and the "one best answer" mentality they create may not be optimal preparation for the ambiguities and uncertainties of real clinical practice. (See Chapter 37, Units of Learning, Not Units of Teaching; Chapter 11, Mirror, Mirror; and Chapter 31, Training to Competence.) In the extreme, national standardized examinations are seen as having become something of an end in themselves. In the conventional scenario, clinical teaching and medical practice are seen as the "hen" that uses the assessment "egg" to produce another hen; as the critics see it, however, what has really happened is that the national examination system has turned things upside down, so that the assessment egg is now using the hen to produce another egg.

Evaluating educational effectiveness and learners' progress at each of the four levels of professionalism presents unique challenges—and unique opportunities. Knowledge assessment is the best established and most widely accepted evaluation technique, probably because the methodologies for measuring knowledge are the most quantitative and the most highly developed. The rigorous, statistical science of psychometrics that has grown up around knowledge assessment now sets the pace for assessment in the other areas of professional life; reliability, validity, generalizability, are now (or now should be) in the lexicon of all assessment techniques. For all its sophistication, however, the assessment of knowledge still presents its own serious challenges. Thus, for example, despite efforts over the years to develop new and better species, the multiple-choice question remains virtually the only "hardy perennial" in the neat and manicured knowledge assessment garden.

Recognizing that knowledge is just the beginning of professionalism, many have also tried to get beyond measuring what doctors know (their knowledge), to measuring what they do (their clinical competence, or skills). Unfortunately, the best of these efforts has been frustrated by both logistic difficulties and the sheer intellectual complexity of the task. Thus, the examination of clinical skills at the bedside was, for many years, a major requirement of American Board of Internal Medicine (ABIM) certification; lack of consistency in both the substrate (the patients and their medical problems) and the technique (the standards used to judge the candidates) led to its demise. Its nonobligatory successor, the Clinical Examination, or CEX, administered during residency training, is widely appreciated for its teaching value. Like its ancestor, however, it has not proved satisfactory as an assessment instrument, in either psychometric or logistic terms (2,3). These shortcomings have led to the development of a new Mini-CEX, a shorter exercise, which is meant to be repeated frequently, and which has already demonstrated substantially greater reliability and generalizability (but not necessarily greater validity) than the previous CEX (4). More on clinical skills assessment later.

Assessing clinical performance is even more of a challenge than assessing clinical skills, and the techniques used in measuring it are varied and ingenious:

- Individual record audits, using implicit or explicit criteria, or more sophisticated methods like "criteria mapping" (5)
- Statistical measures—everything from the way medical records are kept, to the frequency and type of prescriptions written and tests ordered, to the resources used (cost of care)
- Videotaping of individual patient encounters (6)

The results have been tantalizing, sometimes useful, often ambiguous. Increasingly, it is recognized that the challenge of measuring performance won't go away—and some progress is, in fact, being made. Thus, as part of its recertification program, the American Board of Internal Medicine has set about devising a statistically meaningful measure of overall performance for everyday clinical practice using standardized assessments of physicians by their professional colleagues. This assessment tool has already undergone field testing for reliability, although its validity also remains to be established (7). And other groups are now also hard at work developing survey instruments to assess the quality of doctors' clinical performance from the patient's point of view, a critical but almost entirely neglected dimension of performance evaluation (8).

Outcomes assessment is not exactly new, since measures like disease incidence and mortality rate have been with us for a long time. What is new, however, is the ability to measure outcomes over large numbers of patients and providers, and over long periods of time, particularly through the use of large computer databases. Moreover, the need to correct for differences in disease severity and patient characteristics, both of which can seriously confound outcome measurements, is now better appreciated, and statistical techniques are now available for this purpose. Still relatively young, these newer approaches to outcomes assessment are making slow but steady progress, led by groups like the one at Tufts School of Medicine, and are a critical element in the Continuous Quality Improvement effort.

Returning now to clinical skills (competence), the assessment challenge here is to create consistent, statistically reliable test situations (i.e., clinical simulations) for examinees that at the same time are clinically valid—that is, faithful enough to real medical work to measure convincingly the "something beyond knowledge" that is clinical skill. In the paper-and-pencil era, efforts to walk this narrow line led to the development of Patient Management Problems (PMPs), which were, for a time, part of both the American Board of Internal Medicine examination and the American College of Physicians' Medical Knowledge Self-Assessment Program. PMPs boasted good "face validity," but they were extremely difficult to write, were a psychometric nightmare to score, and, worse still, did not convincingly get at the "something" of clinical skills beyond knowledge. The "Cambridge Case," a reformulated successor to the PMP that has been under development for several years, largely in Canada, promises to overcome many of the PMP's limitations, although it is not without its own problems (9). Other hybrid techniques like chart-stimulated recall and live discussions that use standardized written cases and predetermined judgment criteria for responses have fared better as meaningful measures of clinical competence in certain disciplines, particularly in emergency medicine.

Naturally, the advent of microcomputers raised hopes that, at last, it would be possible to develop electronic test cases and scoring techniques sophisticated enough to measure the "something different" of clinical skills, and to do so quickly, cheaply, and conveniently. The Computer Based Examination, or CBX, which has been extensively field tested by the National Board of Medical Examiners, is probably the best developed and best known of these instruments (10). It, too, has presented enormous challenges in both case development and scoring methodologies, and has not had an easy time demonstrating that it measures more than what multiple-choice questions do. Other intriguing microcomputer-based systems are in the works, for example, the hypertext programs, *DxR* from Southern Illinois and *Clinician* from Southern California, and automated case generation by "expert systems" such as *Iliad* and *QMR* , but their place in the clinical skills assessment armamentarium has yet to be determined.

Perhaps the most promising way to assess what doctors do is by using standardized patients—ordinary citizens trained to play the roles of patients with specific problems and to participate in the scoring. The technique works particularly well in assessing the skills of medical interviewing, history taking, and the physical examination, but less impressively in areas of clinical reasoning and management skills. The use of simulated patients is expensive, as well as labor- and time-intensive, but despite these limitations, the technique apparently meets faculty, student, and resident needs sufficiently well that many medical schools and some medical residencies in the United States now include it as part of their standard evaluation systems (11–13). Standardized patients have also been used with impressive effect in medical schools in China and in a variety of other countries as well, both for teaching and for evaluating clinical skills.

In Canada, a major nationwide program is now in place that is designed to assess periodically the clinical skills of all practitioners using a variety of approaches, including simulated patients. By way of contrast, assessment of the clinical skills of practicing physicians in the United States is still just a cloud on the horizon no bigger than a man's hand. The similarities in medical education and practice between the two countries make it likely that the Canadian experience will be important in deciding whether to put together a similar "mosaic" of techniques for assessing the clinical knowledge, skills, performance, and practice outcomes for every practitioner in the United States. What we still don't know, and will need to know, is whether such an assessment package will be seen as necessary, useful, credible, and cost-effective to both physicians and the public—or whether it will simply be seen as the assessment egg yet again using the hen to create another egg.

REFERENCES

1. **Marston RQ, Jones RM.** Medical Education in Transition. Commission on Medical Education: The Sciences of Medical Practice. Princeton, NJ: Robert Wood Johnson Foundation; 1992.
2. **Kroboth FJ, Hanusa BH, Parker S, Coulehan JL, Kapoor WN, Brown FH, et al.** The inter-rater reliability and internal consistency of a clinical evaluation exercise. J Gen Intern Med. 1992;7:174-9.

3. Noel GL, Gerbers JE Jr, Caplow MP, Cooper GS, Pangero LN, Harvey J. How well do internal medicine faculty members evaluate the clinical skills of residents? Ann Intern Med. 1992;117:757-65.

4. Norcini JJ, Blank LL, Arnold GK, Kimball HK. The Mini-CEX (Clinical Evaluation Excercise): a preliminary investigation. Ann Intern Med. 1995;123:795-9.

5. Greenfield S, Lewis CE, Kaplan SH, Davidson MB. Peer review by criteria mapping: criteria for diabetes mellitus. The use of decision-making in chart audit. Ann Intern Med. 1975;83:761-70.

6. Hays RB. Self-evaluation of videotaped consultations. Teaching and Learning in Medicine. 1990;2:232-6.

7. Ramsey PG, Wenrich MD, Caroline JD, Inui TS, Larson EB, LoGerfo JP. Use of peer ratings to evaluate physician performance. JAMA. 1993;269:1655-60.

8. Gerteis M, Edgman-Levitan S, Daley J, Delbanco T. Through the Patient's Eyes: Understanding and Promoting Patient-Centered Care. San Francisco: Jossey-Bass; 1993.

9. Bordage G, Page G. An alternative approach to PMPs: The "key features" concept. In: Hart I, Harden R, eds. Further Developments in Assessing Clinical Competence. Proceedings of the Ottawa Conference on Continuing Medical Education. Montreal: Can-Heal Publications; 1987:59-75.

10. Clyman SG, Melnick DE, Clauser BE. Computer-Based Case Simulations. In: Mancall EL, Bashook PG, eds. Assessing Clinical Reasoning: The Oral Examination and Alternative Methods. Evanston, IL: American Board of Medical Specialties; 1995.

11. Stillman PL, Swanson D, Regan MB, Philbin MM, Nelson V, Ebert T, et al. Assessment of clinical skills of residents utilizing standardized patients: a follow-up study and areas for application. Ann Intern Med. 1991;114:393-401.

12. Gordon JJ, Saunders NA, Hennrikus D, Sanson-Fisher RW. Interns' performances with simulated patients at the beginning and the end of the intern year. J Gen Intern Med. 1992;7:57-62.

13. Anderson MB, Kassebaum DG. Proceedings of the AAMC's Consensus Conference on the Use of Standardized Patients in the Teaching and Evaluation of Clinical Skills. Acad Med. [special issue] 1993;68:437-83.

CHAPTER 27

Severity

The Missing Link Between Disease and Illness

*T*he science of curing has been growing rapidly for about 150 years, and is now exploding with the energy of molecular medicine. The art of caring has been with us as long as there have been people, but the science of caring (which is not as oxymoronic as it sounds), in contrast, is a relatively recent development and continues to evolve very slowly.

Language may be our key to understanding the science of caring. For buried in words is a condensed history of ideas that provides a window onto the conceptual evolution of disease and illness, much as fossils in geologic strata open for us the record of biological evolution. Since language is also the avenue through which we actually implement both the art and the science of caring, we would be well advised to understand that fossil record of ideas.

The language of diagnosis is particularly germane, since in medicine (as elsewhere) we act on the basis of what we believe is going on, and diagnosis describes what is going on in medicine (1). All physicians accept certain everyday expressions such as "streptococcal pharyngitis" as complete diagnostic specifications and, as such, as the very basis of the science of curing. And, indeed, the fossil record of meaning buried in these phrases encompasses the basic elements of our hard-won biomedical model of disease: etiology (the streptococcus organism), anatomy (the pharynx) and pathophysiology ("-itis" = inflammation).

But while these everyday diagnostic descriptions are generally recognized as complete specifications of *disease*, something is missing here.

Where in these syllables is the *patient's* model of "being sick"? What's missing is an expression of the patient's experience of *illness.*

Curiously, the patient's experience of illness was part of the specification of disease in the not so distant past, but has since been lost. Thus, as recently as 1923, the scheme developed by the New York Heart Association for specifying cardiac diagnoses included the fourth element of *function,* in addition to the elements of *etiology, anatomy,* and *pathophysiology* (2). The creators of this classification scheme clearly meant the word "*function*" to connote the impact of disease on a patient's life. And the concept that gives dimension and texture to that impact, and therefore serves as its principal quantitative measure, is *severity.*

Severity, which ranges in degree from nil to fatal, thus turns out to be the element missing from the everyday language of diagnosis; and it is severity that provides the crucial "missing link" between the medical model of disease (etiology, anatomy, pathophysiology) and the patient's experience of illness. This being so, it is clear that it is difficult to give shape to the impact of disease on patients' lives, or to teach the science of caring, without a deep understanding of the nature of severity (3).

There is bad news and good news about severity. The bad news is that severity isn't a single, homogenous concept. For example, when patients refer to an illness as "severe" they are usually thinking of suffering or distress, most often pain (3). In contrast, physicians know very well that severe illness is often present in asymptomatic patients, for example, in patients with silent narrowing of the left main coronary artery or malignancies in silent locations. Severity is, therefore, a subtle and complex mix of elements.

The good news is that, arguably, severity can be well understood as a blend of only four distinct elements: *distress, disability, seriousness,* and *urgency* (see Table 1, "Four Elements of Severity"), which may be described as follows:

- **Distress** is whatever makes the patient feel unwell—pain, shortness of breath, cough, disfigurement, anxiety, you name it; only the patient knows about it for sure.
- **Disability** is interference with function; while patients are often aware of it, others can and must be able to judge it, too.
- **Seriousness** is threat to life; this is most often but not exclusively a perception by medical people.
- **Urgency** is the immediacy of the need for intervention; many people

TABLE 1
Four elements of severity

Element	Information Sources	Example	Measuring Instruments
Distress	Patient	Pain	Introspection, Interview
Disability	Patient, other	Amputation	ADL, etc.
Seriousness	MD, other	Metastatic cancer	APACHE, etc.
Urgency	MD, other	$K^+ = 8.5$	Clinical judgment

can recognize urgency, but that recognition often requires a medically trained eye.

Interestingly, the four elements that characterize *disease severity*—distress, disability, seriousness, and urgency—roughly parallel the four elements used to characterize *disease status* in problem-oriented progress notes—subjective, objective, assessment, and plan—which suggests that the two constructs share a common deep structure or "grammar."

Consider now the following four patients:

- A 28-year-old woman with occasional panic attacks
- A 50-year-old man with mild headache, papilledema, and a blood pressure of 250/140
- A 65-year-old asymptomatic woman eight weeks postmastectomy for breast cancer, with eight out of ten nodes positive
- A 78-year-old woman living alone, who has lost forty-five pounds in six months, is prone to falls, and is increasingly forgetful

Table 2, "Gauging the Elements of Severity," contains a rough-and-ready assessment of the degree to which each element of severity is present for each of these patients, on a scale of 0–4+. Several important features of severity immediately jump out from this crude profile, as follows. First, each element varies independently. Therefore, while every disease contains all the elements, the degree to which each element is expressed depends on the disease and, to some extent, the patient. From this it is clear that a single, lumped "sum" of severity is not helpful in understanding the impact of a disease on any given patient's functional state. Second, strong values, both intellectual and

TABLE 2
Gauging the elements of severity

Element	Panic Attack	Malignant Hypertension	Breast Cancer	Failure to Thrive
Distress	4+	1+	4+	1+
Disability	2+	0	1+	3+
Seriousness	0	3+	4+	3+
Urgency	2+	4+	0	1+

emotional, are attached to each element. These values differ widely among the various participants involved in the care of any given patient—physicians, administrators, patients, families, and others— and these differences are an important clue to hidden sources of the tensions that often arise during care.

Take our patient with panic attacks. During attacks, the patient herself is almost certainly convinced she is dying, and between attacks she dreads their occurrence. We aren't surprised, therefore, when she tells us she believes her illness is "severe." In contrast, physicians know that panic attacks are not a threat to life, and while temporarily disabling, they rarely lead to lasting damage. While physicians will be generally empathetic with her distress, most would not consider occasional panic attacks to be a "severe" disease: two different agendas, hence the potential for major misunderstandings.

Or take our elderly patient who is failing to thrive. Her family finds her inability to function increasingly intolerable; her physician is genuinely concerned that her weight loss represents a serious underlying disease, for example, malignancy. They agree, therefore, that there is a "severe" medical problem here. But when failure of this patient's support system brings her to the emergency room, the hospital staff does not see enough urgency in the situation to warrant admission. For them the problem is not severe—and another potential conflict is born.

The arrival of this elderly patient in the emergency room highlights another important aspect of severity, namely the concept of severity as *resource use*. This is a perspective that defines the severity of a disease by the time, supplies, equipment, and, above all, money consumed in its care. In contrast to the other four patient-centered elements, however, judgments about resource use are made principally by administrators, legislators, payers, economists, and the like, rather than by physicians, patients, or families. The cost of an MR scan is a highly visible example of a resource-based measure of severity, and the commonest unit of measurement is probably still the hospital bill.

Because resource use has become such a compelling issue, the severity of a disease has, unfortunately, been equated increasingly but unknowingly with resource use rather than with the patient's functional state (4). This equation has now become established to a point where severity measurements that are themselves based partly on resource use are used to predict resource use, a circular logic that is open to serious criticism (5). But the flawed logic of resource use as a measure of severity becomes even more obvious through cross-national comparisons. For example, the cost of care for a patient with an acute myocardial infarction in a good hospital in the developing world might be equivalent to $1 per hour, while that for a similar patient in the United States might be as much as $1,000 per hour. Does this mean that a patient's heart attack in the developing world is 1,000 times less severe than in the United States?

There is no argument with the importance of resource use in medical care. But if severity is to occupy its proper niche in medical education, we need to distinguish very clearly between extraneous elements such as economics versus the four elements that make up the human core of the medical concept of severity. If we fail to make that distinction, we risk passing on to our students a distorted, even counterfeit, view of the link between disease and illness. If we keep the distinction clear, we are in an excellent position to link the physician's universe of disease to the patient's universe of illness (6).

REFERENCES

1. **Glenn ML.** On Diagnosis. A Systemic Approach. New York: Brunner/Mazel; 1984:xiii.
2. **Committee on Cardiac Clinics of the New York Heart Association for the Prevention and Relief of Heart Disease.** Requirements for an ideal cardiac clinic and a system of nomenclature. Boston Med & Surg J. 1923;189:762-8.
3. **Cassell EJ.** The Nature of Suffering and the Goals of Medicine. New York: Oxford University Press; 1991.
4. **McMahon LF Jr, Newbold R.** Variation in resource use within diag-

nosis-related groups. The effect of severity of illness and physician practice. Med Care. 1986;24:388-97.

5. **Feinglass J, Martin GJ, Sen A.** The financial effect of physician practice style on hospital resource use. Health Serv Res. 1991;26:183-205.

6. **Davidoff F.** On being a patient. Ann Intern Med. 1996;124:269-70.

CHAPTER 28

Heart and Head

Feeling and Thought in the Teaching of Medicine

*M*edical education is defined principally as an affair of the head, not the heart; its terms are "intellectual, rational, cognitive, orderly," and the like. Yet just under its cool, clean surface lurks a strong current of emotion.

Just occasionally, that underlying emotional (and social) current rises to the surface. Thus, the noncognitive has now begun to influence teaching and learning in certain areas, through a typology for the emotional reactions that influence acceptance and use of information [1,2], for example, and through constructs like self-determination theory [3] and social influence theory [4]. Many influences are undoubtedly at work here, but what has principally kindled the interest of researchers and teachers in such matters is the consistent observation that practice guidelines have little effect on medical practice unless clinicians are also energized to use them by emotional and social forces [5,6].

For the most part, however, this emotional (and social) undercurrent remains unacknowledged in medical education, and when dealt with at all is seen as a negative, something that distorts and distracts from the essentially cerebral tasks of learning. Given the growing concern about the shortcomings of medical education's effectiveness, however, the time is at hand to harness these powerful but nonrational forces to the task of improving clinical practice.

A good place to begin is with the typology of the generic elements of medical practice developed by the distinguished scholar and educator

George Miller. Each element requires an appropriate action, as follows: knowledge, which obviously requires *knowing;* competence, which requires *knowing how;* performance, which requires doing; and desired outcomes, which require *doing well* (Table 1). Certain key emotional states are associated with, hence are important to, learning and practicing each element, as also shown in Table 1. Thus, knowing something depends on *being interested* in it; learning how to do something depends on *believing* it; doing things requires *being confident* in both your knowledge and your abilities; and continuing to do things effectively depends on your *taking satisfaction* in the results.

Being Interested

While it is certainly possible to get knowledge into your head without being interested in a subject, it is intuitively obvious, and now also a well-documented educational observation, that knowledge is absorbed better when you are interested in the subject. Indeed, a major task of continuing medical education is to convert what's good for learners (needs) into what interests them (wants). (See Chapter 34, Continuing Medical Education.) Moreover, there is little question that information that's interesting to a learner, once absorbed, is retained longer than information that's not.

The whole notion of what makes something interesting is, in itself, an interesting subject. "Interest in" something is made up of a variety of component parts, including pleasure, arousal, and dominance (3), which vary with the topic, the presentation, the presenter—and the learner. Thus, some subjects and some presentations seem intrinsically more interesting than others—for example, topics that are neither too simplistic nor too complex, presentations that are neither too monotonous nor

TABLE 1
Generic elements of medical practice

Element of Practice	Action	Associated Emotion
Knowledge	Knowing	Being interested
Competence	Knowing how	Believing
Performance	Doing	Being confident
Desirable outcome	Doing well	Taking satisfaction

too slick. But at its core, interest in something is always in the mind of the beholder. Teachers and learners must therefore share the responsibility for making things interesting. It is also arguably true that the ability to make things interesting is, in itself, teachable and learnable, indeed an essential if neglected skill for both teachers and learners in medicine. (See Chapter 12, The Dilemma of the Uninteresting Patient.)

BELIEVING

Even when you have acquired knowledge about a subject that interests you, it is hard to put that knowledge into practice unless you also believe it—that is, find it credible. Peer review serves as much to enhance the credibility of journal articles as it does to ensure their scientific accuracy; accuracy and credibility are not one and the same. And lectures implicitly tell listeners what information to trust simply by the lecturer's choice of material (a feature of lectures which, at least in some people's eyes, helps compensate for their inefficiency as a way of learning)—that is, selectivity in choosing material to present carries the implication that what the lecturer chose is more believable than what he or she did not.

When practicing physicians avoid implementing practice guidelines, they do so not so much because they don't know about or understand them, but because they don't believe in them. That is, they "distrust guidelines written by so-called national experts," tending rather to "rely primarily on their own experience or colleagues' recommendations in deciding whether to adopt new techniques or interventions" (4–6). To the extent clinicians do trust a specific formal guideline, their trust depends on who produced the guideline at least as much as on its content (5). Moreover, modeling of clinical practices by opinion leaders (who are sometimes referred to in continuing medical education circles as "education influentials") (7) and academic detailing (personal "teaching" office visits to practicing clinicians from nonindustry clinical pharmacologists and pharmacists) (8) are powerful educational interventions. How do these various "educational" techniques gain their particular effectiveness if not by using educators' personal and professional authority to increase practitioners' trust in certain information, much of which the learners often already "know" intellectually?

BEING CONFIDENT

Even knowledge you trust is hard to put into practice unless you are also appropriately confident in your grasp of that knowledge *and* your ability to apply it (your competence). The difference between knowing something and being confident in your ability to use it is like the difference between weather reporters saying "There's a 75 percent chance of rain today" (knowledge) and their saying "I'm only 20 percent sure I know what I'm talking about" (confidence). Ideally, your degree of confidence in your knowledge and abilities would always be exactly "calibrated" to your actual, demonstrated capabilities. All too often, however, people are either overconfident ("one who knows not and knows not that he knows not") or underconfident ("one who knows but knows not that he knows"). (See Chapter 22, Confidence Testing.)

Miscalibration of confidence in either direction can obviously interfere with clinical performance—for example, physicians who get into trouble by assuming they can handle certain problems when, in fact, they really need expert consultation; or at the other extreme, those who are unwilling to manage many simple patient problems without involving a host of consultants. Interestingly, as it turns out, most physicians are overconfident, at least as measured by the quantitative techniques now available for the purpose (9). (This should come as no surprise, given the degree to which decisiveness is rewarded in medicine, and given patients' expectations that physicians will not only know what they need to know but will also have, and convey, confidence in their own abilities.) Equally interesting, however, is the observation that people become better calibrated when they receive feedback that demonstrates their miscalibration. (See Chapter 22, Confidence Testing.)

In light of these observations, it seems only reasonable that achieving a clear understanding of the distinction between knowledge and confidence should be among the most basic goals of medical education. And we all—medical students, residents, practicing physicians, and medical faculty alike—might gain professionally if we were given regular feedback on how well our confidence was calibrated to our abilities.

TAKING SATISFACTION

Finally, even the most interested and confident clinician finds it difficult to maintain a high level of clinical performance in the absence of satisfying, and satisfactory, outcomes. An oncologist, for example, who feels the only satisfying outcome is cure is likely to burn out relatively quickly; one who also takes satisfaction in making terminal illness and death as comfortable and humane as possible is more likely to be able to carry on over long periods of time. And similarly in generalist practice, "the required level of commitment is possible only if physicians find it deeply satisfying to spend 14-hour days" in pursuits that include "the day-to-day commitment, the continual intense encounters with anxious or sick patients and their families, and the requirement to maintain highly technical skills and keep abreast of new knowledge and new techniques" (10).

The nature of satisfaction in medicine is broad, ranging from the intrinsic satisfactions of any job well done, to the professional ones of patients improved or cured, the interpersonal ones of meaningful patient relationships (11), and the extrinsic ones of status, control, and money. Professional satisfaction is an intriguing and endlessly intricate subject, but not one whose importance is widely appreciated or that is well understood, studied, and taught, at least not within medicine.

If, more generally, the emotional and social dimensions of learning are so important, it seems only logical that the heart should occupy a seat at the medical education table along with the head, which is rarely the case. Probably only our psychoanalytic colleagues can answer the question of why it doesn't. Whatever the explanation, both medical education and our patients might be a great deal better off if it did.

REFERENCES

1. **Lipowski EE, Becker M.** Presentation of drug prescribing guidelines and physician response. QRB Qual Rev Bull. 1992;18:461-70.
2. **Greco PJ, Eisenberg JM.** Changing physicians' practices. N Engl J Med. 1993;329:1271-3.
3. **Deci EL, Valelrand RJ, Pelletier LG, Ryan RM.** Motivation and education: the self-determination perspective. Educational Psychologist. 1991;26:325-46.
4. **Mittman BS, Tonesk X, Jacobson PD.** Implementing clinical practice guidelines: social influence strategies and practitioner behavior change. QRB Qual Rev Bull. 1992;18:413-22.
5. **Tunis SR, Hayward RS, Wilson MC, Rubin HR, Bass EB, Johnston M, et al.** Internists' attitudes about clinical practice guidelines. Ann Intern Med. 1994;120:956-63.
6. **Davis DA, Thomson MA, Oxman AD, Haynes RB.** Changing physician performance. A systematic review of the effect of continuing medical education strategies. JAMA. 1995;274:700-5.
7. **Lomas J, Enkin M, Anderson GM, Hannah WJ, Vayda E, Singer S.** Opinion leaders vs. audit and feedback to implement practice guidelines: delivery after previous cesarean section. JAMA. 1991;265:2202-7.

8. **Soumerai SB, Avorn J.** Principles of educational outreach ('academic detailing') to improve clinical decision making. JAMA. 1990;263:549-56.
9. **Christensen-Szalanski JJ, Bushyhead JB.** Physicians' use of probabilistic information in a real clinical setting. J Exp Psychol Hum Percep Perform. 1981;7:928-35.
10. **Mundinger MO.** Advanced-practice nursing: good medicine for physicians? N Engl J Med. 1994;330:211-4.
11. **Suchman AL, Matthews DA.** What makes the patient–physician relationship therapeutic? Exploring the connexional dimension of medical care. Ann Intern Med. 1988;108:125-30.

CHAPTER 29

A Technology for Remembering

Aphorisms and Maxims

*C*lassmates, some twenty-five of us, marking the passage of thirty-five years since we had left medical school, were gathered around the dinner table. The reminiscences began to flow, and in no time at all someone was quoting the Rules of Therapy we had all learned as students, attributed at the time to Robert Loeb, the inspiring (and intimidating) chief of medicine at Columbia in those days:

1. The Golden Rule ("Do unto others . . ").
2. If what you're doing is working, keep doing it.
3. If what you're doing isn't working, stop it.
4. Keep 'em out of the hands of the surgeons.

Now the surgeons in the group weren't about to admit they live by these rules. But all of us, including the surgeons, had to admit that these rules had made a significant difference during our thirty-five years of professional life. For sheer educational staying power, these rules are hard to beat.

We aren't talking mnemonics here—mental tricks, like the hoary "On Old Olympus' Towering Top . . ." beloved of medical students—used for memorizing complicated or confusing material. (Ironically, as time passes, we increasingly can't remember what the mnemonic stands for, even though we can remember the mnemonic itself.) Rather, this is the power of aphorism, which, according to the Oxford English Dictionary, is "a concise statement of a principle in any science," or maxim, "a rule or principle of conduct . . . a precept of morality or prudence expressed in sententious form."

And relative to so much else we learned in our med student days, those legion of things that seemed so important then but are now long forgotten, what educational power it is! It can hardly be an accident that the most effective leaders and teachers in history, from the Buddha and Christ to Mao, Churchill, and JFK, have relied so heavily on aphorisms and maxims, and are remembered particularly for that aspect of their teaching. The term *aphorism* itself (according to the Oxford English Dictionary) originated with the "Aphorisms of Hippocrates" and from there was "transferred to other sententious statements of the principles of physical science and at length to statements of principles generally."

It should be particularly gratifying then to physicians to know that, as a matter of historical record, medicine is a parent and precursor discipline to all of education, at least in this respect. And it seems only fitting, therefore, that aphorisms have been used by great medical teachers in an unbroken chain reaching from Hippocrates though William Osler and Robert Loeb, on to Eugene Stead (whose aphorisms have been collected in a volume called "What This Patient Needs is a Doctor" [1]) and others, right up to the present day.

Like all power, however, the power of aphorisms (and maxims) can be abused. The abuses are mainly of two types. The first is the "literal truth" abuse. This happens when people assume that because an aphorism (or maxim) is true, it is the whole truth. Thus, while any particular aphorism may be compelling, it is also true that for every aphorism there is virtually always a counter-aphorism. "Man does not live by bread alone," is met with "But by bread at least," and on hearing Loeb's Fourth Rule, the surgeon responds "But a chance to cut is a chance to cure." Living by a maxim is frequently the right thing to do, but rigid adherence to any single maxim can get you into big trouble, which may explain why aphorisms and maxims, in medicine at least, are often couched in ironic or self-mocking language.

The second type of abuse is the "borrowed authority" abuse. Aphorisms are expressions of authority as well as of fact and, as such, derive their power from their source as much as from their content. The problem, of course, is that authorities are sometimes wrong, since authority often derives from social or political standing, and personal or even spiritual charisma, as much as it does from knowledge, wisdom, or experience (2). And while the authority of individual experts in medicine still retains a certain unassailable value, it is also the case that the *implicit* (idiosyncratic) expertise of *individual* authorities, whether expressed as aphorisms and maxims, lectures or textbooks, is increasingly complemented—and challenged—by *explicit* (public) and *collective* expertise, as seen in the movement toward evidence-based medicine (3,4).

Moreover, authority alone can't explain all of the educational impact of aphorisms and maxims, since their source is frequently unknown. (Loeb himself is said to have disavowed authorship of the Rules of Therapy, although as students we chose to believe otherwise.) What is it about these "concise statements" that makes them resonate so long in our heads? What are the intrinsic properties of aphorisms that make them stay with us over time? Most importantly, they endure because they capture and reflect deep understandings. For example, the banal-sounding aphorism "Common things are common" which, along with its corollaries "Go where the money is" (a.k.a. "Sutton's rule") and "When you hear hoofbeats, don't think first of zebras," is widely used in medicine, turns out to be a highly memorable and useful expression of Bayes' theorem. This theorem is an abstruse but profoundly important general concept of human information processing that deals with likelihoods, prior and posterior. Few physicians really understand, much less use, Bayes' theorem in its original, quasi-mathematical form, but everyone unwittingly uses it regularly, disguised as an aphorism.

But even deep understandings may pass unnoticed and unused if they are cloaked in ordinary or ugly (e.g., technical) terms. This unfortunate truth was perhaps most clearly recognized by another great medical teacher at Columbia, Dr. David Seegal, who described the variety of ways in which he had transformed the "face repugnance" of crucial precepts into "face value" (5). For example, after many unsuccessful attempts to convince his students of the importance of being able to say "I don't know" on rounds, he learned by chance that this phrase could be stated in early English as "Ic ne wat." He soon discovered that students not only remembered the new form of the phrase and used it frequently, but now in a sense enjoyed admitting their ignorance (the self-mocking tone of the phrase may have helped here). Seegal concluded emphatically that he "would be content to use Sanskrit, Gaelic [mathematical] formulas or even cartoons" as part of his educational armamentarium if that's what it took to get such lessons across.

Seegal's technique of putting a "racing stripe" on everyday teaching is one variant of a more general metamorphosis, the kind that transforms ordinary language into art—what Leonard Bernstein called "the big push" that creates the "super-surface structure" of music and of poetry (6). Thus, the best aphorisms and maxims use the aesthetic and musical properties of language, transforming it in ways that are well known to composers and to poets: repetition, inversion, alliteration, chiasmus (a special form of reversal, as in Kennedy's "Ask not what your country can do for you, but what you can do for your country"), and the like. Examples abound in the aphorisms of medicine, as in

• "Start low, go slow" (the approach to therapeutics in office practice)

• "The person in the family, and the family in the person" (a key to understanding the social context of disease and illness)

• "If it's wet, dry it, if it's dry, wet it; if it's open, close it, if it's closed, open it" (a beginner's approach to dermatology)

• "Diabetes care is most effective when the patient becomes the doctor, and the doctor becomes the consultant" (another of favorite of Robert Loeb)

• "All patients are interesting; some patients are just a little more interesting than others" (the "generalist's creed")

• "A good medical history is a more powerful instrument than a CT scan" (a perspective on the relative value of clinical information sources)

Poetry has been described as "a technology for remembering" (7). Aphorisms are not exactly poetry, but they do manage to "carry meaning beyond the literal, the tangible, beyond the grossly semantic" (in Bernstein's phrase), and thus are metaphors in the original sense of that term (*meta-*, beyond; *pherein*, to carry). It is this "metaphoric leap" that generates the added or inner meaning in music and poetry—and, it appears, in aphorisms and maxims. "It is metaphor which most produces knowledge" says Aristotle. He places metaphor "midway between the unintelligible and the commonplace," an apt description of aphorisms and maxims.

Learning clinical medicine is such a complex process that we deliberately separate learning medical concepts (the development of general mental models) from learning through the "gut-level" experience of direct patient care, a distinction captured by Lee Schulman's exquisite aphorism, "Principles are powerful, but cases are memorable." The beauty of aphorisms and maxims is precisely that they are both.

REFERENCES

1. **Stead E, Wagner GS, Cebe B, Rozear MP, eds.** What This Patient Needs is a Doctor. Durham, NC: Carolina Academic Press; 1978.
2. **Chalmers I.** Scientific inquiry and authoritarianism in perinatal care and education. Birth. 1983;10:151-63.
3. **Evidence-Based Medicine Working Group.** Evidence-based medicine: a new approach to teaching the practice of medicine. JAMA. 1992;268:2420-5.
4. **Paterson-Brown S, Wyatt JC, Fisk NM.** Are clinicians interested in up-to-date reviews of effective care? BMJ. 1993;307:1464.
5. **Seegal D.** The CML^2 reflex for learning on ward rounds. J Med Education. 1962;37:1318-21.
6. **Bernstein L.** The Unanswered Question. Six Talks at Harvard. Cambridge, MA: Harvard University Press; 1976:85.
7. **Pinsky R.** A man goes into a bar, see, and recites: "The quality of mercy is not strained." New York Times Book Review. September 25, 1994. p 15.

PART FOUR

THE SOCIAL, POLITICAL, AND ECONOMIC CONTEXT

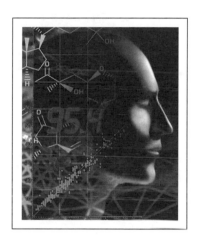

CHAPTER 30

Does Continuing Medical Education Work?

A single instructor lectures and lectures and lectures fairly large groups of . . . people who sit for long hours in an audiovisual twilight, making never-to-be-read notes at rows of narrow tables covered with green baize and appointed with fat binders and sweating pitchers of ice water . . . (1)

P.M. NOWLEN (1)

*D*oes the scenario sound uncomfortably familiar? The image is all too frequently associated with formal continuing medical education (CME). And while not all CME shares this nightmarish quality, much of it does operate in the "update mode" described above in Philip Nowlen's caricature, that is, long linear streams of information presented to passive audiences.

CME is an enormous undertaking, absorbing hundreds of thousands of faculty and learner hours, and hundreds of millions of dollars each year in the United States. To an outsider, an investment on this scale would imply that the value of CME is well established, and that physicians and CME providers alike clearly must also believe this is so. After all, the learners continue to "vote with their feet" (and their checkbooks) for CME; would they do so if it weren't worth something to them?

A good many educators, critics, and researchers have had their doubts. Over the years, they've begun to ask the hard questions, studying the effectiveness of CME in a rigorous, scientifically valid, objective way in an effort to find out whether CME actually "works." After all, doctors are scientists (or so many of us believe). Shouldn't the evidence for the educational effectiveness of CME be just as convincing as, say, the evidence for the effectiveness of a diagnostic imaging technology, or for the therapeutic effectiveness of a drug?

There is bad news and good news from these efforts. First, the bad news. The subject is extremely difficult to study. The methods required are complex, time consuming, hard to control. What outcome do you measure? In the past, the quality of CME programs has all too often been judged by participant satisfaction or financial self-sufficiency; occasionally, it's been judged by the number of facts or concepts participants have absorbed. While more and better knowledge in doctors' heads is without doubt necessary for better practice, measuring increases in knowledge accurately is not easy (witness the enormous psychometric expertise and resources used by the certifying boards and the difficulties they encounter even with all this effort). More to the point, even an accurate measure of CME-related increases in knowledge is hardly a sufficient measure of its effectiveness, in terms of what it is ultimately intended to do: change clinical practices in ways that lead to improved patient outcomes. (See Chapter 26, What Can Doctors Do? and Chapter 6, Commitment for Change.) But as anyone involved with quality improvement programs knows, measuring changes in clinical practices and patient outcomes is even harder than measuring changes in knowledge.

And if you can measure improvements in practice or outcome, how will you know the changes are attributable to a specific education program? Physicians are exposed to a great many powerful forces that could influence their practice patterns: reading, discussion with colleagues, the sheer experience of practice, and the like (2). The effect of any given CME program is, therefore, almost always "contaminated" by these other influences (3), which makes these studies even harder to interpret.

These methodological concerns aside, what the best of these initial studies actually showed was that formal CME programs had no specific, measurable effect on participants' medical knowledge (4). This was particularly true of programs that consisted solely of "predisposing" techniques (i.e., that focused on communicating or disseminating information—Nowlen's knowledge updates). And the more rigorous the study, the less the effect (5). However, critics of this earlier work pointed out that the researchers may have been asking the wrong questions, testing oversimplified hypotheses. It is clear, after all, that practicing doctors learn; they actually do change their practices (2). They learn to do new procedures, to handle new diseases and new ways to handle old ones; they learn to use new drugs, and new and better ways to use old ones. The more important question, therefore, may be what *does* really bring about the changes, not what CME doesn't do or why it doesn't do it (2).

As an aside, failure of formal CME to detectably change clinical practices may not be all bad. Concepts and practices that seem right today turn out to be wrong or inappropriate tomorrow: Witness the evolution of peptic ulcer from a stress-related disease to an infectious one. To some degree, therefore, healthy conservatism has a role to play in medicine, and patients may be better off in some respects if doctors don't jump at every new fad or trend handed down by faculty experts (6). Looked at this way, exploration and questioning of the evidence, debate, and discussion are important aspects of CME, more important, perhaps, even than the dissemination of expert or "received" knowledge. (See Chapter 15, Ideals and Motivations.)

The good news is that the research continued; the methods improved; the evidence accumulated (7–9). And while the task is far from complete, the data indicate that CME does indeed work: Doctors do change their practices in response to CME programs, particularly when those programs involve "enabling" strategies (on-site interventions within practices that support or facilitate the sought-after changes—for example, patient education activities or so called "academic detailing"), "reinforcing" strategies (mainly reminders and feedback), or, most impressively, multifaceted single interventions, or programs that combine all three strategies (predisposing, enabling, and reinforcing). Moreover, it is also clear that formal CME not only changes physician practices, it also improves patient outcomes, despite there being less evidence that this is so (7–9).

Data showing that formal CME can work are important, but they represent only the numerator in the equation. The broader question is "CME is effective relative to what?" or, stated differently, "What proportion of all effective practice-improvement interventions does formal CME contribute?" This question can really only be answered by looking at the problem the other way around, that is, by examining the changes physicians make in their practices, then by figuring out what fraction of those changes is attributable to formal CME. The work of Fox and colleagues (2) addressed exactly this question in a serious and systematic way, and found that formal CME (organized programs or courses with faculty-specified learning objectives) played at least some role in two thirds to three fourths of the changes made by physicians. Thus, while formal CME contributes to continued professional improvement, it is by no means the only important contributing factor. Reading journals, consulting with colleagues, teaching, and other activities—informal rather than formal CME—may actually be at least as important as formal CME, if not more so, in bringing about these improvements (see Chapter 37, Units of Learning, Not Units of Teaching, and Chapter 7, Lifelong Learning) (2,4,8–10).

In retrospect, CME was for a long time the principal instrument for maintaining and improving the quality of patient care, although it wasn't thought of in those terms, since the concept of quality improvement hadn't yet been introduced. Indeed, while "continuous quality improvement" and formal, explicit practice guidelines are the most recent arrivals on the quality improvement scene, CME has quietly been providing physicians with its own informal and idiosyncratic variety of practice guidelines for years. Indeed, all of CME is in a sense practice guidelines—less explicit, official, or "perfect," perhaps, than the newer variety, but flexible, meaningful practice guidelines nevertheless. And while the newer, more formal species of practice guidelines would seem a priori to be more compelling because they are produced and endorsed by groups rather than by individuals, and are often (but not always) grounded more firmly in the evidence, the data so far indicate that, for all their promise, "practice guidelines, when used alone, [are] not effective" (4).

Formal CME therefore still potentially has a major role to play in quality improvement, particularly if it can successfully move away from its heavy reliance on the passive knowledge transfer or "predisposing" strategies embodied in lectures and the techniques of knowledge update and come to grips with issues of competence (working skills such as medical interviewing, case management, counseling, procedures) and performance (the complex, interwoven, personal and situational "on-the-job" factors that determine whether competent physicians actually work up to their potential).

In sum, CME works. Under the newer competence and performance models, it could work even better, although more sophisticated measurement techniques, including self-assessment and possibly even rigorously validated feedback from patients, will be required in order to understand the impact of these new models. Developing the full potential of these newer models will not be easy, cheap, or simple; but then, few things worth doing in medicine are.

REFERENCES

1. **Nowlen PM.** A New Approach to Continuing Education in Business and the Professions. New York: Collier Macmillan; 1988:23.
2. **Fox RD, Mazmanian PE, Putnam RW.** Changing and Learning in the Lives of Physicians. New York: Praeger; 1989.
3. **Goldfinger SE.** Continuing medical education: the case for contamination. N Engl J Med. 1982;306:540-1.
4. **Davis DA, Haynes RB, Chambers L, Neufield, VR, McKibbon A, Tugwell P.** The impact of CME: a methodological review of continuing medical education literature. Evaluation and the Health Professions. 1984;7:251-83.
5. **Sibley JC, Sackett DL, Neufeld V, Gerrard B, Rudnick V, Fraser W.** A randomized trial of continuing medical education. N Engl J Med. 1982;306:511-5.
6. **Burnum JF.** Medical practice a la mode. How medical fashions determine medical practice. N Engl J Med. 1987;317:1220-2.
7. **Davis DA, Thomson MA, Oxman AD, Haynes RB.** Evidence for the effectiveness of CME. A review of 50 randomized controlled trials. JAMA: 1992;268:1111-7.
8. **Davidoff F.** CME in the U.S. Postgrad Med J. 1995;72:536-8.
9. **Davis DA, Thomson MA, Oxman AD, Haynes RB.** Changing physician performance. A systematic review of continuing medical education strategies. JAMA. 1995;274:700-5.
10. **Manning PR, DeBakey L.** Medicine: Preserving the Passion. New York: Springer-Verlag; 1988.

CHAPTER 31

Training To Competence

 ⌒

So Crazy It Might Just Work

S ome students learn faster and more easily than others. But if variability is such a basic fact of educational life, why are most medical education programs the same length for all comers—the late bloomers and the fireballs alike? True, an occasional medical student or resident who gets too far behind his or her classmates is asked to take an additional course or rotation, or occasionally is even required to repeat a year's work before moving on; the opposite—moving learners ahead as soon as they've mastered the material—is practically unheard of. But on the face of it, the present system, in which all students are moved forward in lock-step formation, is not an efficient use of the limited time, effort, and dollars available for educational purposes, from anyone's point of view—students, faculty, or institutions. Can it be that medical trainees are getting more education than they really need? Is there such a thing as too much of a good thing in medical education?

Efficiency has never been a big issue in education, particularly the medical variety. For one thing, the conventional wisdom has it that you can never learn too much about a subject as enormous as medicine, especially when the lives and health of patients are at stake. It would seem churlish, at the very least, to suggest stripping down medical education for the sake of mere efficiency. Besides, how would you define educational efficiency? And how would you measure it?

All the same, in this era of growing demands and shrinking

resources, it isn't unreasonable to rethink the question of efficiency. One obvious place to start is with the possibility that medical trainees should stay in programs only as long as it takes them to meet some predetermined educational goals, then move on to the next step: training to competence, as it is referred to in the trade. While this concept at first seems outlandish, even a bit crazy (particularly in medicine where the curriculum is packed to bursting), the evidence suggests that when it comes to length, medical learning is, in fact, quite forgiving. During both World Wars, for example, medical school training was significantly shortened without demonstrable detriment to the skills and subsequent careers of the periods' graduates. In the 1960s and 1970s, the flush of enthusiasm for graduating all those additional doctors so desperately needed to maintain the country's health (O tempora, O mores!) also produced a number of three-year medical school programs, again without apparent harm to the trainees or to their patients. In the present day, several quasi-experimental, condensed programs of the Ebert-Ginzberg type have started up, allowing at least a selected few of the most capable students to move through the system at an accelerated rate; reports from the field on these programs have so far been favorable (1,2).

Psychometricians have, of course, made their living all along from the variability of student learning, and since educational testing is expensive in terms of time and money, they have been forced to care about test efficiency. As the power and flexibility of testing have grown and the understanding of test operating characteristics has improved, a variety of creative and increasingly efficient testing techniques have therefore evolved. It is now clear, for example, that as long as a test is sufficiently reliable, you can confidently identify higher-scoring students by first using a short version of that test, thus saving time, sweat, and tears for both students and faculty. Only the smaller number of students who don't do well on the initial short version need then go on to more extensive testing, which establishes their performance level with greater accuracy and confidence. Now if psychometricians working in their microcosm can do it, why can't the rest of the educational system follow suit? Why not simply define a set of increasing levels of competence we want students and residents to achieve at the various stages of professional development, assess their achievement frequently and regularly against these criteria, then send them on their way to the next level of training once they meet each standard?

And why stop with students and residents? Physicians in practice learn—from reading, from courses, but most of all, from the experience of taking care of patients and reflecting on that experience. Common sense, plus much anecdotal information, tells us that the competence of seasoned clinicians grows with time. (We should probably call such professional development "working toward higher competence" rather than "training to competence," since they are not, strictly speaking, in training, and there is no easily identified upper bound to the competence level they are trying to achieve.) In light of the obvious growth of so many physicians into expert, even master clinicians over their years in practice, the observation that practicing clinicians' scores on repeat board examinations tend to decrease over time seems strange, even paradoxical (3). The decline in scores is generally attributed to the erosion of practitioners' competence, but that explanation seems thin. Could it be that board examinations, in fact, simply don't measure the more important elements that make up *advanced* clinical competence? Weak test validity, rather than deterioration of skills, might just be what accounts for much of the observed change in practitioners' scores.

In pondering the possibility of developing a more efficient, streamlined medical education system, then, what emerges is the need above all to define and measure high-level competence. The first step here would be to recognize that when we talk about measuring or training to "competence," we are using the term loosely. We are talking about an enormously complex, multilayered entity, yet to be named, that includes knowledge (knowing), competence (knowing how) and performance (doing), not to mention critical but even more subtle personal, professional, and humanistic dimensions (4). (See Chapter 24, The Right Hand of Claude, and Chapter 16, Why Is Teaching Valued Less Than Research?)

Second, we must also acknowledge that we are still not very good at measuring medical competence—the very thing medical practice most needs, and therefore the most important thing that medical education can produce at this high level. Yes, many medical schools have their own assessment programs that serve the lock-step system well enough; yes, we have widely accepted standardized national licensing examinations; and yes, we have a highly credible system of specialty board certification (in which eligibility requirements are probably as important as the written examinations). But despite the best efforts of many capable people over many years, the clinical skills evaluation tools essential for creating a tailored medical education system simply don't exist, at least not with the degree of sophistication and at the high-stakes level of validity and reliability suitable to the purpose.

Indeed, the creators of existing clinical assessment systems would be the first to admit that, while the existing instruments measure some meaningful elements of competence, they fall short of measuring the essential totality of advanced medical competence. We know, for example, that roughly 40 percent of medical interns can pass the written internal medicine Board Certification examination (5). But no one would seriously claim on that basis alone that the interns who pass are ready to go right out and practice medicine.

Training to competence would also need to face a third and daunting reality, that of logistics. For how could you ever plan an education program—hire faculty, line up patients, make up class or lab schedules, or put together "coverage" for clinical services—if you were never quite sure how many students or residents would be arriving for your course or rotation, how long they would be staying, or when they would leave? The mind reels at the thought. Moreover, a fluid system like this would deprive students and residents of the opportunity to learn from each other, develop mutual support systems, and experience the camaraderie and spirit of a class that stays together as it moves along through the program. A train-to-competence system would repeatedly break up the naturally formed groups of learners, forcing medical students and residents to learn and to function more on their own, much like the graduate students in other disciplines do already.

A fourth reality of training to competence would be the need to determine what level of competence students would have to achieve before ending one course and moving on to the next. A system in which they needed only to perform at a lowest common denominator level, consistent with safety but nothing more, would be neither practical nor credible; it might be expected to lead over time to mediocrity, superficiality, and a self-reinforcing downward spiral of eroding goals (6). By contrast, a system in which all students were expected to demonstrate extremely high levels of performance before continuing on could promote the development of a more elite profession overall. But "raising the bar" this high would be possible only at the cost of sacrificing those students who couldn't clear these extreme hurdles but who would have been competent, solid practitioners had they been allowed to complete their training. A standard somewhere in the middle, while not a perfect standard, thus seems to be the only viable option. It would certainly be more acceptable than the "low ball" alternative, although it would not, by itself, support the pursuit of excellence. Specialty certifying boards have struggled for decades with this quandary, moving slowly but progressively from the elite standard of their early years to the present standard in the middle range. Neither standard has ever seemed entirely satisfactory, and perhaps there really isn't an optimal one.

All of this is not to say that more streamlined, tailored systems, systems that train to competence, might not happen in the fullness of time. It's just that the obstacles are presently formidable enough to make the idea of developing them seem a little crazy—as were once the ideas of democracy, moon shots, computers . . . .

REFERENCES

1. **Ebert R, Ginzberg E.** The reform of medical education. Health Aff (Millwood). 1988;7:5-38.
2. **Thompson JS, Haist SA, DeSimone PA, Engelberg J, Rich ED.** The accelerated internal medicine program at the University of Kentucky. Ann Intern Med. 1992:116:1084-7.
3. **Ramsey PG, Carline JD, Inui TS, Larson EB, LoGerfo JP, Norcini JJ, et al.** Changes over time in the knowledge base of practicing internists. JAMA. 1991;266:1103-7.
4. **Schumacher CF.** Validation of the American Board of Internal Medicine written examination. A study of the examination as a measure of achievement in graduate medical education. Ann Intern Med. 1973;78:131-5.
5. **Levinson W, Kaplan C, Williams G, Clark WD, Williamson P, Lipkin M Jr.** What is an expert in medical interviewing? J Gen Intern Med. 1993;8:713.
6. **Senge PM.** The Fifth Discipline. The Art and Practice of the Learning Organization. New York: Doubleday; 1990:383-4.

CHAPTER *32*

In the Vanguard

Teaching Medicine in the Community

[with Susan Deutsch, MD]

*I*nternal medicine is practiced primarily in ambulatory settings. Approximately 95 percent of all physician encounters occur in the offices of doctors in individual and group practices, and hospital out-patient settings (1). The National Ambulatory Medical Care Survey reports that there were approximately 96 million ambulatory visits to internists in the United States in 1990 (2). Despite these simple realities, the hospital care model has remained at the core of clinical education in internal medicine for many decades, for both students and residents. More specifically, the patient occupying a hospital bed has been virtually the exclusive subject of internal medicine teaching, ever since hospitals began to be seen as the ideal environment for exposing trainees not only to the clinical manifestations of human disease but also to the excitement of scientific medical practice.

It was not always so. Before the rise of the hospital as a middle-class institution, the teaching of medicine in the United States happened primarily where it was practiced, in patients' homes and in physicians' offices (3), and learning was primarily by apprenticeship. Hospitals were extensions of almshouses for the poor and destitute, and were where students and residents went to see the chronically and incurably ill, the odd and exceptional (4). But toward the last half of the nineteenth century, beginning with the advent of scientific medicine, gaining momentum from the academic model at the Johns Hopkins Medical

175

School, and consolidated by the 1910 Flexner Report, the hospital became the temple of scientific medicine, and hospital-based teaching has remained the traditional model ever since.

At the same time, the spectrum of internal medicine practice has gradually shifted, particularly during the last half-century, away from care of acute disease, largely of infectious origin, and toward chronic disease, much of it related to high-risk behavior and to the process of aging. In parallel, the "curing" model of internal medicine of the 1950s is being increasingly replaced by the "managing" model of the 1990s. The availability of increasingly sophisticated diagnostic and therapeutic technologies has also meant that many important patient management decisions formerly made inside the hospital now occur outside it.

Throughout these last five decades, internists who practice outside the walls of the academic teaching centers have known a professional universe that has remained well hidden from those inside academic walls. It comes as no surprise to these community-based physicians that 95 percent of care takes place outside the hospital, since they are the ones who deliver that care. They understand that their practice is inseparable from the many threads that make up the fabric of community life—the schools, the nursing homes, the health officers, the sports teams, the local economy and its trades and occupations, the other practitioners in the area—in sum, the local culture of their community's neighborhoods, its myths and traditions, its civic pride, and its secrets.

Toward the end of the 1980s, the rate of change in medical practice began to increase exponentially. Escalating costs and an administrative typhoon that has swept away old forms of economic risk and swept in integrated care systems have created inpatient services populated increasingly by the critically ill, those affected by long-term high-risk behavior, and those admitted for invasive procedures. And, certainly, AIDS has contributed to the transformation as well. Inpatient settings have thus become increasingly high-tech, rapid-fire, narrowly focused, and complex places in which to work, teach, and learn. And while inpatient settings have for a long time been an incomplete educational environment, the mix of patients and diseases and the philosophy and organization of care in today's acute care hospitals are rapidly becoming even less appropriate than they were in past decades as the central focus for the training of today's and, particularly, tomorrow's internists.

The effect of such heavily inpatient-oriented training on the knowledge, skills, and attitudes of those already committed to careers in internal medicine is one thing. Its effect on student career choice is quite another. Many of today's internists can identify one or more practicing doctors who years ago both inspired their choice of career and served as models for professional behavior. Today, few internal medicine trainees have significant exposure to "real live" practicing internists of that kind, since most students are taught by busy internal medicine residents and by hospital-based, full-time (salaried) academic faculty; the role of the "voluntary" faculty has diminished profoundly. This concern is *not* simply nostalgia for the good old days that probably never existed; it is a matter of facing up to hard, cold realities.

One important result of these many and complex changes is that medical students and residents learn a great deal about internal medicine as a *discipline,* but few medical students or residents have ever seen or learned about internal medicine as a *practice.* And the practice of internal medicine—that is, first-contact, continuing, personal care; moving between the office and the hospital; and serving as primary care doctors and as consultants—in brief, "putting it all together" into a clinical professional life—can really only be learned from internists who live that professional life in the community. Hospital clinic experience teaches certain aspects of ambulatory medicine, but community-based practice requires a variety of important generic professional competencies that are particularly important in that setting: time management, use of community resources, intimate working relationships with practicing colleagues, and the realities of developing and managing an office-practice team, to name a few.

Moreover, practitioners in several follow-up studies have made it very clear that their hospital-based residency training fell short in a variety of important areas—dealing with psychosocial problems, geriatrics, rehabilitation medicine, taking sexual histories, nutrition counseling, sports medicine and office orthopedics, office ophthalmology, gynecology, and dermatology, and the like—as preparation for community-based practice. Managed care organizations also complain that it takes a year or two to "untrain" internists newly graduated from traditional, hospital-based training, and to initiate them into the realities of practice in integrated, largely ambulatory care systems. Clearly, then, a substantial training-practice mismatch exists in internal medicine.

A second result of the many changes in the practice environment is increasing distress among those excellent community-based internists whose professional self-image includes teaching ("doctor" comes from a root meaning "teacher"). And a third result is that the real careers of most internists (i.e., those in the community), long perceived only dimly by students, have now become virtually invisible. The consequent loss in understanding about, and the attractiveness of, community-based careers, particularly those of generalists, has contributed to a continuing decline in the numbers of U.S. medical students who choose those professional pathways.

Response to the erosion of careers in community-based internal medicine has been slow in coming. In the early 1990s, however, departments of medicine in a number of medical schools, along with many of the major internal medicine organizations, began developing programs to facilitate the use of internal medicine practices in the community as a logical and high-quality site for clinical teaching. In so doing, these groups expect to

- Change the nature and improve the quality of clinical education of both students and residents
- Increase the visibility and attractiveness of internal medicine as a career, thereby increasing the number of students choosing careers, particularly generalist careers, in community-based internal medicine
- Support practitioners through increased opportunities to teach, learn through teaching, and be recognized for their teaching contributions
- Develop the mechanisms for effective medical student and resident mentoring
- Evaluate the effectiveness of community-based practices as teaching sites

One group specifically dedicated to this task is the American College of Physicians' Community-Based Teaching Task Force. Working closely with and through the College's Governors, the task force has concentrated its efforts on putting together "packages" of print materials—on logistics, faculty development, curriculum, evaluation—to support both practitioner-teachers and medical school department chairs, deans, and clerkship directors. Faculty development workshops—interactive, hands-on, working sessions—have been a second major initiative of the group. The intent has been to catalyze the development of a teaching resource that will be as valuable to students, and as important to medical schools and residency programs, as inpatient teaching services have been in the past, if not more so. The expectation is that development of this resource will, at the same time, create teaching opportunities that are as satisfying to the practitioners in the community as the other aspects of their professional life. All agree that such programs must be rigorous, thoughtful, organized. They are, after all, up against a rigorous and unforgiving tradition of hard science on the inpatient side that will be only too ready to see community-based teaching as soft, irrelevant, a waste of time. They must, therefore, like Caesar's wife, be beyond reproach; they will require the best thought and concerted effort of those inside the walls of academe and outside; and above all, they can't afford to fail.

Community-based teaching, long on the periphery of career development in internal medicine, is emerging into the vanguard. It will need to move quickly and well, however, or events will certainly pass it by.

Please contact Dr. Deutsch for further information about the Community-Based Teaching Project: Susan Deutsch, MD, American College of Physicians, Independence Mall West, Sixth Street at Race, Philadelphia, PA 19106-1572. (215) 351-2573.

REFERENCES

1. **Boufford JI.** Changing paths and places for training tomorrow's generalist. Clinical education and the doctor of tomorrow. In: Proceedings of the Josiah Macy, Jr. Foundation National Seminar on Medical Education, Adapting Clinical Medical Education to the Needs of Today and Tomorrow. June 15–18, 1988. Gastel B, Rogers DE, eds. New York: New York Academy of Medicine; 1989.
2. **Schappert SM.** National Ambulatory Medical Care Survey. 1990 Summary. Vital and Health Statistics of the National Center for Health Statistics. April 30, 1992.
3. **Ludmerer KM.** Learning to Heal. The Development of American Medical Education. New York: Basic Books; 1985.
4. **Rosenberg CE.** The Care of Strangers: The Rise of America's Hospital System. New York: Basic Books; 1987.

CHAPTER 33

Guidelines and Continuing Medical Education

G uidelines are hot. The Institute of Medicine has thrown its ponderous weight behind them; Washington's newest health bureaucracy, the Agency for Health Care Policy and Research, has put millions of dollars into them. Most medical specialty societies are developing at least a few; insurers, managed care organizations, and medical think tanks are hard at work on them; even in Canada, guidelines are being taken seriously.

Historically, what triggered the sophisticated process of guideline development was the quantitative documentation of an old and simple observation: doctors' practices vary (1). Once this had been shown in black and white, it was a short step to the conclusion that, if a given, middling rate of use of a given practice was desirable, then the highest rates might represent overuse, while the lowest rates might mean some patients were being deprived. The next logical step was to develop a way to narrow the range of variation: to set standards—guidelines, practice parameters—that defined the outer (upper and lower) bounds of acceptable practice. Guidelines thus evolved originally from the best tradition of medical professionalism; that is, they put a new spin on the old and continuing drive to optimize care, although their application has since developed distinct overtones of cost containment (1).

But guidelines are, in essence, doing the same thing that medical education, including continuing medical education (CME), has always done: guiding and improving clinical practice, bringing it closer to some "expert" standard, and, in the process, making it both more effective and efficient. (See Chapter 35, Managing Messes.) Looked at this way, medical schools and graduate medical education programs can be seen as institutions that generate gigantic sets of practice guidelines for students and residents. And journals, textbooks, consultants, and live CME programs have for a very long time provided guidance—and guidelines—by which practicing doctors refined their clinical skills, and a species of semi-formal standards against which they measured their clinical performance.

So why the fuss all of a sudden about the "new" practice guidelines? What makes them different from the guidelines that are implicit in traditional medical education? The Institute of Medicine has defined practice guidelines as "systematically developed statements to assist practitioner and patient decisions about appropriate health care for specific clinical circumstances." (A specific example is "ambulatory ECG monitoring is useful in evaluating selected patients with symptoms possibly caused by arrhythmias" [2].) But this definition is also an excellent description of most medical education, so it doesn't help much in distinguishing the two. In fact, the nature of formal practice guidelines varies widely—from proposals from individual experts, to consensus statements from groups, to rigorous, quantitative, evidence-based recommendations—depending on who makes them and why. And, of course, education programs vary even more widely, from print self-assessment programs developed by groups, to lectures by individuals, to highly interactive panel discussions among authorities. (See Chapter 35, Managing Messes, and Chapter 11, Mirror, Mirror.) Despite all this variability, on careful scrutiny it is possible to discern consistent differences between guidelines and education, as follows:

- Guidelines aspire to national standards, whereas education frequently incorporates regional, local, and personal standards
- Guidelines are arrived at through a collective intellectual process; education is, for the most part, generated by individual faculty
- Guidelines are officially sanctioned by professional groups and organizations; education carries with it the personal authority of single experts
- Many guidelines are created through explicit, data-driven processes, often quantitative (the "systematically developed statements" of the Institute of Medicine definition); education depends more heavily

on subjective, implicit thinking—expert opinion and clinical judgment—much of it nonquantitative

- Guidelines are "summative," that is, they serve as explicit standards (rules) by which performance is judged (the "appropriate health care" of the Institute of Medicine definition); education tends more to be more "formative," that is, it consists of information (principles) on "how to understand, how to diagnose, how to manage." (See Chapter 11, Mirror, Mirror.)

- Most guidelines are couched in broad, general terms, applicable to defined groups or cohorts of patients (the "specific clinical circumstances" of the Institute of Medicine definition); education is more frequently directed to the management of widely differing individual patients

In a recent comprehensive study of the information used to guide clinical practice, Forsythe and colleagues concluded that physicians need information of several sorts—formal, informal, general, and specific—in the course of their daily work (3). Practice guidelines clearly conform to a defined category of "formal-general" information, that is, "general procedures accepted throughout medicine." While education also employs some "formal-general" information, it depends even more heavily on information that is "informal-specific" and "informal-general," much of it local. Indeed, it is the informal and specific properties that make medical education uniquely effective, for, as Forsythe and colleagues have noted (3),

> Empirical studies of the ways in which human beings make sense of information in a variety of real-world contexts show that informal, specific knowledge is what enables individuals to apply formal, general knowledge.

> Local knowledge is the link between the universal and the specific, between the textbook or journal article and the formulation of a treatment plan for a particular patient.

Clearly, guidelines should now be included on the list of "universals," along with textbooks and journal articles.

Guidelines and education thus express two basic characteristics of medical information, its "formal-general" versus its "informal-specific" properties, respectively, much as sensitivity and specificity express the two principal operating characteristics of medical tests. And just as the properties of tests are reciprocal (i.e., the sensitivity of a given test decreases as its specificity increases), the more broadly medical information applies to groups or populations, the less it applies to a specific patient. David Eddy has described the analogous reciprocal relationships found in cost-effectiveness analysis (4). That is,

> If a category [of treatment] is too highly aggregated [i.e., includes the treatments that apply across many patients and conditions], it is virtually impossible to develop an accurate estimate of its effectiveness or costs. . . . Furthermore, if you do manage to come up with an estimate of the benefit for a highly aggregated category of treatments and indications, the result would not apply accurately to every [individual] treatment/indication in the broad category, which would lead to many erroneous conclusions.

Thinking about all this, it is tempting to conclude that "guidelines are guidelines and education is education, and never the twain shall meet." That view is, of course, simplistic: Informed clinical practice needs both, in much the same way that medical tests need an appropriate mix of sensitivity and specificity, although the need for one may outweigh the need for the other, depending on the specific testing situation. In like fashion, guidelines without education remain "formal-general" abstractions whose everyday clinical relevance and utility are limited (5); education without guidelines remains "informal-specific" advice whose consistency and credibility are limited. It seems likely that as the experience with guidelines development and dissemination grows and the process becomes more sophisticated (6,7), and as medical education, including CME, continues to be tied increasingly to national data standards (8), the two disciplines will move closer to each other; each will borrow from, blend with, and balance the other. At this point, however, we are far from knowing how best to bring guidelines and education together, and it seems likely that the challenge of moving between the general and the specific in the care of patients will always be with us.

REFERENCES

1. **Audet M, Greenfield S, Field M.** Medical practice guidelines: current activities and future directions. Ann Intern Med. 1990;113:709-14.
2. **American College of Physicians.** Ambulatory electrocardiographic (Holter) monitoring. Ann Intern Med. 1990;113:77-9.
3. **Forsythe DE, Buchanan BG, Osheroff JA, Miller RA.** Expanding the concept of medical information: an observational study of physicians' information needs. Comput Biomed Res. 1992;25:181-200.

4. **Eddy DM.** Cost-effectiveness analysis. Is it up to the task? JAMA. 1992;267:3342-8.
5. **Tunis SR, Hayward RS, Wilson MC, Rubin HR, Bass EB, Johnston M, et al.** Internists' attitudes about clinical practice guidelines. Ann Intern Med. 1994;120:956-63.
6. **Hadorn DC, McCormick K, Diokno A.** An annotated algorithm approach to clinical guideline development. JAMA. 1992; 267:3311-4.
7. **Eddy DM.** A Manual for Assessing Health Practices and Designing Practice Policies. The Explicit Approach. Philadelphia: American College of Physicians; 1992.
8. **Antman EM, Lau J, Kupelnick B, Moskeller F, Chalmers TC.** A comparison of results of meta-analyses of randomized control trials and recommendations of clinical experts. Treatments for myocardial infarction. JAMA. 1992;268:240-8.

CHAPTER 34

Continuing Medical Education

Wants and Needs

*I*f we ask cigarette smokers what they want, they might tell us "Lower tar, better filters, less harsh tobacco, lower cost," and the like. If, on the other hand, we ask nonsmokers what smokers need, we will probably be told they need to stop smoking.

When it comes to physician education, the difference between wants and needs can be equally impressive. For example, if asked, doctors might say they want to learn about the latest in angiotensin-converting enzyme inhibitors, but the doctors' colleagues (not to mention their staff and patients) might tell us they really need to learn to get better at talking with patients.

The lesson here is that educational wants are not necessarily the same as educational needs: Wants are subjective, and can be defined only by the learners themselves; needs are defined objectively, by others, for example, or on the basis of data. Taking this logic to its extreme, it might even be argued that learners are among the *least* reliable sources of information about what education should deal with. Medical schools, for example, assume that medical students have no way of knowing what they need to know and the schools' faculties therefore pay little attention to the students' educational wants. (The prescriptive philosophy of medical schools, incidentally, runs counter to a fundamental principle of adult learning, that is, that learners' interests should define what it is they will be learning. This contradiction, curiously enough, is rarely pointed out, although it may have contributed to the develop-

185

ment of problem-based learning in medical schools.)

When physicians reach their practice years, however, the assumption is made that they really *do* know what they need to know, and that these needs determine their educational wants and interests. In a sense, this must be true: who else if not the physicians in the trenches themselves can know what they have to deal with every day, hence what they need to know more about and do better? This is the assumption that underlies the established standards for formal CME programs in the United States. Indeed, one major shibboleth of the CME accreditation process is *needs assessment*. Thus, Essential #2 of the Accreditation Council for Continuing Medical Education requires that "the sponsor shall have established procedures for identifying and analyzing continuing medical education needs and interests of prospective participants."

Unfortunately, like most thinking in this area, this Essential doesn't distinguish clearly between educational needs and wants. Even the English language doesn't help much here, despite the two distinct words for the two concepts, since the dictionary defines a "want" as "something needed" but also as "something desired," while a "need" is defined as "a wish for something that is desired," but also as "a situation in which something is required." Besides, there is the very practical problem that assessing educational wants is much easier than assessing needs, so much so that the concept of "needs" is no longer thought of as being unique and unto itself, but is simply folded into the concept of "wants." Ask doctors what they want to learn and they'll tell you, and whatever they tell you is, by definition, right. The term used for this activity in CME is therefore "needs assessment," never "wants assessment," even though the process almost exclusively looks at what physicians *want* to know.

In contrast, truly assessing educational needs means deciding who else to ask: colleagues? administrators? nurses? patients? all of the above? It means figuring out how to ask them, and how to interpret the information they provide, which is a rigorous and demanding task if it is done right (1). It means looking for other, more "objective" data, such as the results of examinations (self-assessment or other), medical outcome studies, or practice-derived information, all of which are more complex, more difficult, and more expensive to obtain. It is not really a surprise, therefore, that even though we may have decided that needs is the more important of the two, we tend to fall back on assessing wants.

What's more, even at their best, the methods for assessing educational needs and wants leave much to be desired. As noted, wants assessment in particular focuses on knowledge (wanting to understand more about ECGs, for example, or about viral hepatitis), since knowledge is so much easier to find out about, even though the real quality problems may lie with shortcomings in competence or performance. (See Chapter 35, Managing Messes.) Moreover, powerful, well-defined psychological biases—for example, the tendency to recall cases that are recent even though they may be less important (recall bias)—can easily affect the responses to surveys of educational (particularly knowledge) wants (2). Wants assessment is also limited by the basic methodological problem that doctors (or anyone else) can't want something they don't know about, even though they would want it if they did know. And finally, wants assessment suffers from peoples' universal bias toward learning in areas where they are already knowledgeable, which is more rewarding than being pushed into areas where they feel awkward or naive; no one likes the "eat your vegetables, they're good for you" approach to education.

Educational needs, in contrast, are increasingly defined by national standard-setting bodies, through the development of practice guidelines, consensus statements, and the like. (See Chapter 33, Guidelines and Continuing Medical Education.) But while a standards approach makes sense in principle, it cannot be expected to work well in practice unless it takes both time and place carefully into account. For example, by the time an education program based on a guideline that recommends a new practice is ready to go, most doctors may already have learned about the practice and adopted the recommendations, making the program redundant (which, of course, raises the important question of how they came to learn about the practice in the first place). At any point in time, moreover, the adoption of a guideline may vary widely from place to place, so that educational need varies according to geographic location (3).

Finally, as noted, the most important educational needs often lie in areas of competence or performance, which are less well defined than specific knowledge content, and much harder to measure. A recent well-known example highlights the difficulty. Several well-publicized instances of misdiagnosis of uterine cervical cancer led legislators some years ago to conclude that the performance of staff in the clinical laboratories was inadequate, that is, that the technicians who read the Pap smears were making errors because they were insufficiently trained. This quasi–needs assessment, in turn, contributed to the passage of the Clinical Laboratory Improvement Act (CLIA), a complex, expensive, and onerous bureaucratic regulatory mechanism. However, a later, more careful assessment of the problem concluded that, while the quality of technicians' reading wasn't ideal, the principal difficulty was that clinicians were collecting inadequate specimens. The benefits of CLIA are very much open to question; an educational rather than a regulatory remedy based on the first assessment of "needs" therefore would have been equally likely to miss the mark.

An important contribution of the current continuous quality improvement (CQI) approach has been to demonstrate that the complex, tightly knit care systems in which doctors practice are powerful determinants of performance, and hence of the type and quality of care provided. The data generated by high-quality CQI programs also force us to acknowledge that many of the performance problems that lead to less-than-optimal outcomes result from inadequate or malfunctioning care systems rather than from an individual doctor's (or nurse's, or administrator's) lack of knowledge or deficient competence. CQI has thus taught us that educational needs may in fact be *system* needs as well as *individual* ones. Not surprisingly, detailed, data-driven needs assessment, both educational and operational, that draws on many sources of information, is a key part of the CQI process.

In the last analysis, responsiveness to both the educational wants and needs of doctors makes sense. Studies that have looked at the question empirically have found that formal CME programs based on identified physician learning needs and wants are more effective in bringing about changes in practice than those that aren't (4). And there is not much sense in creating even high-quality programs directed at critical educational needs unless doctors also want them, since most formal, organization driven CME programs simply can't survive unless learners are willing to pay for them. (Industry's contribution, which makes up roughly half of all financial support of formal CME, introduces an additional potential problem altogether, namely, the concern that education programs designed to meet the needs and wants of companies, which are substantially commercial, may not address the most important professional needs and wants of the participating physicians.) (See Chapter 36, Continuing Medical Education and Health Care Reform.)

Our current ways of assessing educational needs and wants, including the important contributions of CQI, are still clumsy and inefficient, and the need for new and better assessment techniques is therefore very clear. In this connection, the low-cost, detailed, highly specific, practice-based documentation of educational wants and needs built into the

Canadian Maintenance of Competence system is highly attractive; it deserves a great deal of attention and support. (See Chapter 7, Lifelong Learning.)

Moreover, many individual articles in the medical journal literature regularly specify educational needs identified by the authors, who are usually in an excellent position in the medical community to know where their colleagues fall short. Unfortunately, since these articles are not marked with a uniform identifier (e.g., a Medical Subject Heading [MeSH] term), they must still be identified by hand searching, which is both laborious and inefficient. Given the well-established capabilities of electronic literature searching, it is extremely attractive to consider the possibility of retrieving at the click of a mouse all the recent published papers that document educational needs in a specific medical area—an important opportunity for potentially fruitful collaboration between the private sector (the CME leadership) and the government (the National Library of Medicine).

Most importantly, the health care system as a whole can't afford the time, effort, or dollars to undertake CME it doesn't need. For all its imperfections, needs and wants assessment can only get more important as time goes by, however we do it.

REFERENCES

1. **Epstein K, Laine C, Farber NJ, Nelson EC, Davidoff F.** Patients' perceptions of medical practice: judging quality through the patients' eyes. Am J Med Quality. 1996 (summer).
2. **Kahneman D, Slovic P, Tversky A, eds.** Judgment Under Uncertainty: Heuristics and Biases. New York: Cambridge University Press; 1982.
3. **Kosecoff J, Kanouse DE, Rogers WH, McCloskey L, Winslow CM, Brook RH.** Effects of the National Institutes of Health Consensus Development Program on physician practice. JAMA. 1987;258:2708-13.
4. **Davis DA, Thomson MA, Oxman AD, Haynes RB.** Changing physician performance. A systematic review of the effect of continuing medical education strategies. JAMA. 1995;274:700-5.

CHAPTER 35

Managing Messes

Three Models of Continuing Medical Education

*A*ll professionals, including physicians, don't just solve problems, they manage messes.

But how do physicians learn to do that? And does our present continuing medical education (CME) help them to learn how? Present-day CME consists overwhelmingly of lectures, with a small admixture of seminars, discussion groups, and print self-assessment programs. Their objective is to update the medical knowledge in physicians' heads by presenting large amounts of biomedical facts and concepts, along with expert guidance in clinical practice, with the expectation that absorption of more knowledge of this kind leads to better medical outcomes. Unfortunately, this "knowledge update model" of CME is only moderately effective and minimally efficient as a way of increasing physician knowledge and improving clinical practice. (See Chapter 30, Does Continuing Medical Education Work?, and Chapter 37, Units of Learning, Not Units of Teaching.)

Medicine might therefore be taken to task for focusing its continuing education efforts so narrowly. Medicine, however, is not the only discipline in which "the information-intensive, short-course update is overwhelmingly the characteristic continuing education response," as pointed out by Philip Nowlen, who has made a career of studying continuing education across the professions (1). By way of explanation, Nowlen suggests that the update model, in addition to expressing "the traditional American love of new gadgetry and dread of being caught up in a fad past its prime," reflects lack of familiarity with the concepts and practices of adult education (2). Moreover, the update model reflects the prevailing view of the structure of knowledge and the way professionals "know." That is, "professionals feel 'most professional' when they are applying a research-based technique or protocol . . . when their problem solving is firmly grounded in the world of certainty, stability, and rigor." Unfortunately, Nowlen continues, knowledge updates "view professionals as if they were at the passive end of a series of mediatory steps, each at increasing distance from the world of 'real' knowledge."

The knowledge update approach has found a certain measure of success in improving simpler and more narrowly focused practices, such as prescribing. And then there is, of course, the extremely practical reality that update-model CME is much less labor intensive, less demanding of faculty skill, experience, and commitment, than the more intensive forms of education, such as mentoring, tutoring, and direct clinical supervision. But given the "messes" of clinical medicine—that is, given its extremely complex and intensely pragmatic nature—the greater concern here is that the update model simply ignores the concepts and practices of experiential learning (i.e., the practicum approach) (3), which is the principal method by which people learn to manage messes (4). But if professionals' unique and most challenging role is, in fact, managing messes, then the distance of the update model from those "real-world" tasks predicts that facts and concepts absorbed in the knowledge update model will not have much useful effect on professional performance. This, in fact, appears to be the case (see Chapter 30, Does Continuing Medical Education Work?, and Chapter 37, Units of Learning, Not Units of Teaching) (5), a disconnect sometimes referred to as the "knowledge-performance gap." The gap is no laughing matter, but the whole situation does bring to mind the story about the man who lost his keys down at the corner where it was dark, but looked for them in the middle of the block where the light was better.

Confronted with the limitations of the update model and the widespread existence of the knowledge-performance gap, a number of educators decided about twenty years ago to move continuing education out of its deeply worn knowledge update groove by taking on the much tougher issue of how to make people more competent. They began to create a new working definition of competence by teasing out the essential elements required for managing messes in dry but precise terms such as "the acquired intellectual, attitudinal and/or motor capabilities derived from a specified role and setting . . . an integration or synthesis

of behavioral objectives as well as some elements of covert behavior."
Becoming competent clearly requires more than knowledge. But what?

A full understanding of competence, it appears, requires knowing
exactly what elements make up a professional's job. For example, in
1976, a committee of pharmacy practitioners set out to examine what
pharmacists do all day. They began, not surprisingly, with the assumption that pharmacists' principal activities consist of the measuring, formulating, compounding, and dispensing of drugs; they ended, surprisingly, with the realization that pharmacists primarily spend their time
interacting with patients. The result, ultimately, was a shift from traditional update model continuing pharmacy education, which had
focused almost exclusively on pharmaceutical chemistry, drug action,
formulation, and the like, to competence model education directed at
learning to handle counseling, education, support, and the other important aspects of pharmacist–client relationships.

In the twenty years since this effort began, much thought and effort
have been devoted to dissecting out the essential elements of jobs, the
building blocks of competency, in a variety of businesses and professions. The result has been lists of descriptors such as "new roles preparation," "critical skills of mind," "socio-emotional maturity," "logical
thought and the ability to conceptualize," and "entrepreneurial abilities." On the one hand, therefore, it has become increasingly clear that,
while competence obviously requires professional knowledge, the
requirements of competence go far beyond knowledge. On the other
hand, it has not proven easy to translate the deeper understanding of
job functions thus obtained into educational experiences that effectively improve competence.

Despite all the difficulties, these concepts have become the basis for a
"competence model" of continuing education. Readings, films, discussions, role playing, videotaping of learners in action, as well as the whole
repertoire of "reflection-in-action" used by skilled coaches (3), including
academic detailing, opinion leaders, audit with feedback, reminders and
other systems, have emerged as the principal techniques and instruments
of this model. And the specific competencies now being tackled under
the model include a variety of complex behaviors such as medical interviewing, counseling, clinical management, and diagnostic workups. (See
Chapter 26, What Can Doctors Do? and Chapter 14, Medical Interviewing.) As predicted, competence-model education turns out to be
both more expensive and labor intensive than its update-model counterpart, and more often pushes learners out of their so-called "comfort

zone." There is relatively little hard information as to its effectiveness, but the few data that do exist suggest that continuing medical education in the competence mode is considerably more powerful than update-model education as an agent of professional change (5).

To confound the situation, it is clear that even highly competent professionals don't always manage messes effectively, that is, *perform* effectively on the job if, for example, they are in the wrong job, or if they are placed in an incompetent or chaotic organization, or if pressures from outside their job are excessive. As Nowlen points out, "The most serious flaw in the competence approach is its implicit assumption that performance is entirely an individual affair." This leads the competence model—logically, if too narrowly—to an exclusive focus on individual workers. Thus was born the performance model of continuing education, which includes the knowledge and competence elements of job performance, but broadens its concerns to include an intricate "double helix" in which the characteristics and competencies of individual practitioners are intimately entwined with the cultural and social networks of the organizations in which they work.

If continuing education in the performance model sounds complicated, it is. If it also sounds familiar, that may be because the performance model shares many elements with Continuous Quality Improvement (CQI), the increasingly powerful system for managing messes that has evolved outside of, and in parallel with, continuing education over the past fifty years. CQI, which is found nearly everywhere these days, focuses on individuals working within complex human systems; on process and outcomes data; and on team development (6), aspects of professional function that obviously include but go far beyond the issues of individual competence.

In medicine, CQI has been applied principally in hospitals and managed care systems, rather than in the personal care of individual patients in individual physician practices. In contrast, CME has been viewed as the major instrument of quality improvement for individual practitioners. But in theory, at least, many of the principles of the population-based approach to quality improvement embodied in CQI are just as relevant to personal, one-on-one care of patients as they are to large complex care systems; conversely, the knowledge, competence and performance models of CME have many applications in larger systems. These two approaches have met in a middle ground that now includes techniques such as *practice guidelines, clinical pathways, needs analysis, outcomes analysis,* and the like, and disciplines such as *clinical epidemi-*

ology, decision analysis, and *evidence-based medicine.* While still unfamiliar to many, these concepts and techniques are slowly and progressively making their way into both medical education and CQI. (See Chapter 33, Guidelines and Continuing Medical Education.)

And, increasingly, the realization has grown that CQI itself is in fact a powerful form of CME, performance-model CME, at that. Curiously, with that realization has come some concern within the CME community that CQI could even beat CME at its own game, not necessarily a bad thing since it may serve as a wake-up call to CME. An alternative and more optimistic view is that, while performance-model CME and CQI began separately, they will ultimately converge. Managing messes is a serious challenge that continuing education has not yet met head-on, so the outcome of such a convergence would likely be to everyone's benefit; at the very least, it's likely to be interesting.

REFERENCES

1. **Nowlen PM.** A New Approach to Continuing Education in Business and the Professions. The Performance Model. New York: Collier Macmillan; 1988.
2. **Knowles MS.** The Modern Practice of Adult Education. Chicago: AP Follett; 1980.
3. **Schön D.** Educating the Reflective Practitioner: Toward a New Design for Teaching and Learning in the Professions. San Francisco: Jossey-Bass; 1988.
4. **Kolb DA.** Experiential Learning. Experience as the Source of Learning and Development. Englewood Cliffs, NJ: PTR Prentice Hall; 1984.
5. **Davis D, Thomson MA, Oxman AD, Haynes RB.** Evidence for the effectiveness of CME. A review of 50 randomized controlled trials. JAMA. 1992;268:1111-7.
6. **Berwick DM, Godfrey AB, Roessner J.** Curing Health Care. New Strategies for Quality Improvement: A Report on the National Demonstration Project on Quality Improvement in Health Care. San Francisco: Jossey-Bass; 1990.

CHAPTER 36

Continuing Medical Education and Health Care Reform

Over the years, much has been made of industry's financial support for continuing medical education (CME)—an amount estimated to be somewhere between $100 million and $200 million per year—and its potential for distorting education to serve promotional purposes. But as the smoke has (intermittently) cleared on this issue, the failure of the medical profession itself and of society in general to provide adequate, stable funding for CME has increasingly emerged as a fundamental problem underlying many of the present difficulties in industry–CME relationships.

For reasons beyond the scope of this discussion, people are generally reluctant to pay for education—witness the salaries of teachers versus those of neurosurgeons. And while future physicians (and their families, who foot the bills) see medical school and residency as worthwhile investments, practicing physicians have been much less willing to pay for CME out of pocket. This reluctance is, in part, responsible for the financial "vacuum" into which flow dollars from industry, creating a kind of self-reinforcing or vicious cycle: The availability of industry support reinforces the reluctance to pay, and reluctance to pay creates the opportunity for more industry support. The dynamics of this cycle, over the years, have created a system of support for CME that is now tightly locked in, one that will be very difficult to change.

The turmoil over CME funding is particularly salient in light of the continuing debate over the inadequacies of the U.S. health care system.

Few of the proposals for reforming the system have included education as a prominent part of their reform strategy, and CME has been particularly conspicuous by its absence here. Those proposals that have dealt with education at all have focused principally on the relationship of education to manpower, and the related issues of funding for medical school and residency training. The assumption therefore seems to be that we can achieve a new and better medical care system, *and* not break the bank, by using economic, regulatory and legislative mechanisms alone. Education does not figure as a credible instrument for bringing about or sustaining any of these changes. In fact, federal legislators are quite aware that doctors earn a great deal, and consequently clearly agree with medical students and their families that medical education is a good investment. The result, not surprisingly, is the legislative perception that spending public funds for medical education is highly discretionary, one of the things that is most dispensable when it comes to reducing the drain on the public purse.

Now it would be naive to assert that the legislative pundits are all wrong, and that medical education must become a "big gun" in the effective, and cost-effective, reform of the health care system. Yet at the same time there is a disturbing degree of naiveté in the legislative position that says the public interest in medical education is so limited that public funding should in no way be committed to direct support of the medical education system. It is true that a decision to go into medicine is a purely personal one; no one forces you to go to medical school, so it does make sense to expect medical students to continue to assume a substantial part of the financial burden of their initial training. Even here, though, medical students are the very doctors who will soon be making the clinical decisions that not only determine the quality of health care but who also control 80 percent or more of the annual spending of a trillion health care dollars, 50 percent or more of which come directly out of the public pocket. Leaving aside the indirect subsidy of medical student and resident education that occurs through public funding of research grants to faculty (a dubious benefit from the strictly educational point of view), it therefore does make sense that at least some medical student and resident educational funding be publicly derived, especially if that funding can go directly to the support of high-quality teaching.

But the naiveté of "hands-off" legislative thinking on this issue is particularly at fault in its failure to distinguish the fiscal issues surrounding initial training (i.e., medical students and residents) from those related to the continuing education of practicing doctors. In contrast to the student and resident situation, the investment in practicing doctors is a "sunk cost," that is, it has already been made. These practicing doctors *are* the people who are already delivering the medical care; we therefore have no choice *but* to be sure they are making the most effective *and* cost-effective clinical decisions if we are to have a medical system that produces the best possible care and does so without breaking the bank. Here is where continuing medical education enters the reform picture, for while it is true that physicians improve their practices to a limited degree in response to educational leverage, the data clearly show they make more significant and lasting improvements in clinical decision making in response to internal, self-determined forces, supported by educational input, than they do in response to external, regulatory pressures, that is, legislative or regulatory "sticks" and economic "carrots" (1). (See Chapter 30, Does Continuing Medical Education Work?)

In fact, physicians resist noneducational leverage; compliance with regulatory pressure tends to be mechanical and perfunctory. It may also be true that noneducational leverage results in inflexible, arbitrary, "cookbook" medicine unless it is tightly coupled with the kind of flexible, appropriate, smarter practice that can be achieved through education, that is, CME. Pulling back funds or withholding them from continuing physician education and development as a way to make up financial deficits is therefore a short-sighted and misguided strategy, in a sense much like eating the seed corn: it may assuage a present financial hunger, but it risks much more serious professional and, ultimately, fiscal malnutrition in the not-so-distant future.

Health care system reform and CME thus need each other, but how can the two be linked? Recent experiments along these lines in Great Britain and Canada may provide some clues (2). Based on the experience there, it may not be unreasonable to suggest a plan for the United States that would provide every licensed U.S. physician with a supply of CME vouchers each year. These vouchers could be used only for certain designated purposes, for example, as tuition for accredited CME courses, subscriptions for peer-reviewed journals, and the like. Ultimately, it might be appropriate to allow physicians to use them only for educational experiences or instruments shown objectively to be effective, much as third-party payment for medical services is increasingly determined by the demonstrated effectiveness of those services. A focus on educational effectiveness would not only be likely to improve practice quality and efficiency but would also drive the development of research that is so badly needed to demonstrate which education programs are effective and why. Physicians might be encouraged to pursue CME more actively if they received their vouchers only after actually completing a certain amount of CME each year. And unless physicians maintained a certain level of CME activity over time, they might not continue to receive vouchers at all.

At the same time, it seems only right to ask physicians to pay some of the related costs of CME out of pocket (e.g., travel, lodging, and income lost from practice). This is all the more logical because at least some of those ancillary dollars go to the support of industries other than CME itself, making it difficult to justify using general funds for that purpose. Moreover, as things now stand, many of the Category 1 credits are assigned for live courses. These not only require travel, hotel, and living expenses but also incur direct CME costs that are about ten times higher per credit hour than the costs of other, more efficient types of Category 1 CME, such as self-assessment programs (about $30 versus $3, respectively). Requiring continued physician accountability for ancillary costs would thus maintain the pressure to develop more CME that, like self-assessment programs, is efficient as well as effective. Of course, if they wanted to, physicians could pay for CME in excess of the amount covered by the vouchers.

Importantly, these vouchers would *replace* reimbursement dollars to physicians, not *add* to them. The cost of vouchers therefore would not increase the overall cost to third-party payers, be they the federal government, the private sector, or some combination. Instead, the voucher mechanism would channel moneys that are now spent entirely as discretionary dollars into obligatory funding for CME, creating a stable base of support that does not now exist. With support like this, CME program directors could at last leave off the endless scramble for survival and turn seriously to the business of long-term planning; to the developmental work needed to create the next generation of innovative, highly effective education programs.

A voucher plan that provided only $1,000 of dedicated funding annually per physician would buy a lot of high-quality CME for the 550,000 physicians in the United States. The advantages? This amount would go a long way toward reducing the heavy and sometimes inappropriate dependence on CME funding from industry; it would not cost more money (save for some administrative costs for distributing vouchers); it would commit to CME less than one one-thousandth of the total dollars currently spent on health care ($550 million out of nearly

$1 trillion); and most important, as suggested above, it has the potential for substantially improving both the quality of clinical practice and its cost effectiveness.

The disadvantages? Physician incomes (and nonfinancial rewards) being as great as they are, there will be those who argue that doctors themselves, rather than the public, should continue to pay the full freight for their own continuing education. And then there is always the concern that whoever pays the piper calls the tune; that is, spending controlled by a large central bureaucracy runs the risk of becoming an instrument of political and social policy that is far removed from or, even worse, antithetical to its original, intended educational purpose. It may be wise, therefore, to counter this universal tendency to seize and maintain power, by parceling out voucher funding through "block grants" directly to geographic regions, states, or accredited CME organizations, to be used for defined and universally agreed-on purposes but administered as each agency sees fit.

And would such a conditional withholding of funds be just another hidden tax? Perhaps so, in a very limited sense, but definitely not more so than the withholds now widely imposed on physician income by managed care organizations. And unlike those withholds, which provide direct financial incentives to ration medical services, a CME voucher withhold only provides an incentive to stay current, deepen understanding, improve clinical practices—in short, become a better educated and more capable physician—arguably a more socially desirable outcome than those resulting from practice-related withholds.

The winds of reform change in intensity and direction. But the issue of CME support will remain the same whether reform comes from a centralized system of universal access or from integration of services and management of service capacity in a free market. In either case, a health care system that claims to be not only effective and efficient but also intelligent must recognize education as a central, not a peripheral, element.

Would a voucher be a worthwhile investment? Many would argue it's a better investment than $550 million spent on more laboratory testing, for example, or on more invasive procedures. And, since such a system could well begin to pay for itself in a reasonable time through more appropriate care and cost savings, it can even be argued that we can't afford *not* to make an investment of this kind in CME, as an integral part of smart health care system reform.

REFERENCES

1. **Fox RD, Mazmanian PE, Putnam RW.** Changing and Learning in the Lives of Physicians. New York: Praeger; 1989.
2. **Murray TS, Dyker GS, Campbell LM.** Characteristics of general practitioners who did not claim the first postgraduate education allowance. BMJ. 1991;302:1377.

CHAPTER 37

Units of Learning, Not Units of Teaching

～

Toward a Rational Continuing Medical Education Credit System

*T*he current system of defining and awarding CME credit has for many years been taken for granted as a necessary part of the CME landscape. Recently, however, its rationale and its impact have come under increasing scrutiny. More specifically, the recognition is growing that formal, lecture-type teaching, the kind that makes up most Category 1 credit, is favored over learner-documented activities not because of any particularly compelling evidence that it is the more effective form of education, but rather because it is easily organized, documented, and controlled. In the words of Dr. Dennis Wentz, Category 1 credit dominates the CME system because it promotes ". . . what bureaucrats like: evidence of an attendance slip!" (1). There are even those skeptics who suspect that organized, formal, lecture-style teaching prevails largely because this format best serves industry as the vehicle it needs for getting its messages across to physicians.

Why even bother thinking about all this credit business? On the surface, at least, the credit system seems more like an epiphenomenon than a central part of the CME enterprise. But it would be a mistake to write CME credit off too lightly, for as most educators (and students) know well, credit and evaluation systems are powerful "drivers" of education. Indeed, they are viewed in some quarters as being responsible for major distortions of the entire medical education system (2).

The current situation, briefly, is this. CME credit is available in two varieties: Category 1 and Category 2. Category 1 credit is awarded for

201

"documentable and sponsor-verifiable education." In principle, Category 1 credit can be assigned to many types of medical learning. In practice, the vast majority of Category 1 credits are assigned for formal, didactic, live CME programs of the lecture or seminar type, although a few individual learning activities such as self-assessment programs also receive Category 1 credit.

Category 2 credit is "everything else," that is, "the entire range of other education verified by the physician-participant." Category 2 contains a wide variety of personal learning activities not designated as Category 1, that is, not centrally documented, including reading medical journals (above a certain amount), electronic medical literature retrieval, and quality improvement activities. Medical teaching, medical writing, and presentation of papers and exhibits, as well as courses designated as Category 2 by accredited CME sponsors, make up another group of Category 2 activities.

This system produces several ironies. First, as discussed earlier (see Chapter 30, Does Continuing Medical Education Work?), the evidence suggests that the kind of knowledge update, or "predisposing," educational activity that generates most Category 1 credit is minimally effective, if at all, in improving clinical practices and patient outcomes (3). Indeed, it is now clear that the changes physicians make in their clinical practices are driven substantially by forces other than formal, organized education programs (4). It is particularly ironic, therefore, that the type of tailored and self-directed individual learning for which Category 2 credit is awarded comes a good deal closer to embodying the principles of effective adult learning than most formal Category 1 programs. Adult learning—sometimes referred to nowadays as "andragogy," to distinguish it from the way children's education, or "pedagogy," is usually conducted—is rooted in the interests and experiences of the learners, involves learners actively in the learning process, and depends on ongoing self-assessment with continuing feedback (5).

These reflections only underscore the irony that Category 1 credit is widely considered the gold standard in CME. That is, this category carries nearly all of the authority required for maintaining hospital staff credentials, state licensure (approximately half of all states require physicians to obtain formal CME credits, largely Category 1, to maintain their license to practice), and the like. Category 2 credit is generally discounted as being of secondary, even trivial, importance, with the result that most physicians don't even bother to claim credit for the many activities that could count in this category.

Certainly, as physicians we should be accountable for our continuing education, and to this end, some measure of the quality of that education against a national standard, as well as some documentation of our learning and of consequent improvement in our practices, are necessary and appropriate. Unfortunately, it appears that the need for "evidence of an attendance slip" dominates CME to the point where educational effectiveness and priorities have become distorted in the process. Even more unfortunately, documentation of participation in Category 1 CME, which is, after all, its major presumed advantage over the self-documentation of Category 2 credit, is sometimes honored more in the breach than the observance, much to the occasional delight of investigative reporters.

From this perspective, the current CME credit system is not only irrational, but probably also creates perverse rewards in the sense that the less effective activity gets the greater recognition. In a more rational system the two CME credit categories would be reversed. That is, active, adult-learning–type CME activities such reading, consulting with colleagues, searching the literature, teaching, writing—those things, in short, which physicians and their patients very likely benefit most from, and which appear to be the source of most high-level lasting improvements in practice and patient care—would be rewarded with Category 1 credit. (See Chapter 7, Lifelong Learning.) They would also, therefore, become the gold standard for hospital privileges, licensure, and the like. Passive, knowledge-based, "update-type" courses would be in Category 2.

The time has come, therefore, to rethink the CME credit system from the ground up. As noted, reversing Categories 1 and 2 might be more rational, but such a simple, arbitrary exchange begs the underlying question of the utility of documentation in the first place. More importantly, accepting that switch as a sufficient change would ignore an even more fundamental problem with the current system, namely, that it is based on units of teaching (i.e., the amount of exposure to a teaching activity), rather than on units of learning (i.e., the amount of information sought and obtained). The whole purpose of CME is, after all, to increase the quality and quantity of what physicians learn. The amount that is taught (or the amount of time spent being taught) often, unfortunately, has little to do with the quality and quantity learned.

A more rational alternative than switching the names and the status of the present credit categories, therefore, would be to replace the current two-category system with a unitary system that rewards units of learning (things learned, competencies gained) rather than units of teaching (e.g., hours spent). Under this new arrangement, all activities that generate explicit knowledge-seeking activities, particularly those that, in turn, actually lead to the acquisition of new information, would receive some kind of credit. These activities could include participation in formal courses, lectures, or seminars; the use of self-assessment programs; reading journals; electronic literature searches and computer-based learning; performing and using consultations, teaching, writing, and the like. It might be reasonable to specify an appropriate mix or balance of such activities that would be acceptable within a given period of time.

To deal with the issue of public accountability, physicians would be required under this system to keep a log of the problems they investigate, the questions they ask, and the activities they undertake to find the answers, much in the way they now keep patient records or procedure logs. They would be required to share these learning records periodically with accredited CME "guidance" organizations, whether those be state medical societies, professional organizations, medical schools, or other organizations. The role of these organizations would be to validate the logs, document the effectiveness of this form of CME credit, and work with physicians to continuously improve it. Could such a system work? The Royal College of Physicians and Surgeons of Canada has recently implemented a system very much like this one which, despite a number of predictable growing pains, has functioned very well (6,7). (See Chapter 7, Lifelong Learning.)

Keeping additional records is not exactly how most of us would like to spend our precious discretionary time, but physicians already comply with the need to document many activities that are far less rewarding to themselves, and less important to their patients, than their own learning. Electronic log books now make it relatively easy to keep track of units of learning, which can be documented at whatever intervals are most convenient (e.g., weekly) and at a level of detail that "satisfies" rather than provides mathematical certainty. Moreover, since physicians would control both the learning itself and its documentation more completely than they do now, enthusiasm for a new unitary system like the one described is likely to be much greater than when controls are imposed, seemingly arbitrarily, from outside (4).

Finally, the question remains whether such a unitary, self-documented CME credit system would pass muster with those outside the profession to whom we are accountable. This is a more difficult question than it looks. On the one hand, physicians are trusted every day with the most sensitive information from their patients, with potent therapies, with decisions about life and death. Why shouldn't they be trusted to document their own self-improvement? The available evidence indicates that physicians are, in fact, highly conscientious in providing documentation of this sort (8). On the other hand, physicians are fallible, and they are no longer trusted automatically. The better question, therefore, is not whether a unitary, self-documented system would be completely above reproach, but whether it would be an improvement over the present one. It's hard to believe it would be worse.

REFERENCES

1. **Wentz DK.** Continuing medical education at a crossroads. JAMA. 1990;264:2425-6.
2. **Marston RQ, Jones RM.** Medical Education in Transition. Commission on Medical Education: The Sciences of Medical Practice. Princeton, NJ: Robert Wood Johnson Foundation; 1992.
3. **Davis DA, Thomson MA, Oxman AD, Haynes RB.** Evidence for the effectiveness of CME. A review of 50 randomized controlled trials. JAMA. 1992;268:1111-7.
4. **Fox RD, Mazmanian PE, Putnam RW, eds.** Changing and Learning in the Lives of Physicians. New York: Praeger; 1989.
5. **Knowles MS.** The Modern Practice of Adult Education. Chicago: AP Follett; 1980.
6. **Royal College of Physicians and Surgeons of Canada.** The maintenance of competence program. Ann R Coll Phys Surg Canada. 1993;26(Suppl):S3-53.
7. **Evans I.** Canada's style of continuing medical education. Lancet. 1995;346:1093.
8. **Stross JK, DeKornfeld TJ.** A formal audit of continuing education activity for license renewal. JAMA. 1990;264:2421-3.

CHAPTER 38

Education, Patients, and the Public

While doctors accept in principle the professional obligation to educate patients and the public, it is probably the obligation most often honored in the breach. Our shortcomings in this are not to be taken lightly, since our patients tell us that the giving of information is high on the list of things that matter to them. More specifically, the American College of Physicians (ACP) recently asked over 1,000 patients and their internists to rank the potential determinants of the quality of care in office practice. Patients ranked "receiving information" second in importance out of ten major dimensions of care; their physicians ranked "giving information" sixth. Moreover, patients are very clear that they primarily want to get that information directly from their physicians, and in this they may also differ from the physicians themselves. In the ACP study, for example, patients ranked a physician's personal skill in answering questions and explaining medical matters as one of the ten most important practice characteristics out of a list of 125, but the very same patients ranked the availability of printed health education materials in the waiting room last on the list.

The distance between what patients and their doctors think about the value of patient education calls for explanations. Several possibilities come to mind.

To begin with, there are the externalities. Educating the public about medicine is substantially a nonacademic, nonprofessional, even a commercial, pursuit. In fact, much of the best, and best-known, "health" education is produced by nonphysician journalists, authors, scholars, and commentators. For its own reasons, industry has joined enthusiastically in the business of public education, from food companies interested in convincing the public that their products promote good health, to the pharmaceutical industry, which justifies direct-to-consumer advertising of prescription drugs largely on educational grounds.

Then there's the inconstant reaction of the public on the issues of health and disease. On the one hand, people can't seem to get enough information about medicine and health—but on the other, they frequently react with anxiety, sometimes to the point of hysteria, to the latest medical news. Add to this the confusion the media create because they have difficulty interpreting the uncertainties of medical science, not to mention their habit of exploiting controversy among researchers (1), and the area of patient and public education seems like something to stay away from.

Then there is the hard reality of time. Physicians' time in this era of managed care has become a precious commodity, and educating patients takes time. Pressure on physicians to see more patients in less time thus only increases the tension around the obligation to inform and educate patients.

To be sure, some of the problem also has to do with lapses inside the profession itself. Doctors are probably not as good at public and patient education as they are at other parts of their job, which is hardly surprising since acquisition of these skills is a low priority item during their training. This means doctors tend to skirt the task since, like everyone else, they prefer to do the things they do best. Besides, while public education may look easy, it's actually quite difficult and demanding: it requires physicians to think as much from the patient's point of view (how it feels to be sick) as from their own (how disease works), not a simple undertaking. (See Chapter 27, Severity.) Patient and public education also requires physicians to use language in a specific and carefully controlled way, which differs sharply from the way they are trained to use it among themselves (2).

But the professional tensions that surround public education run deeper than the difficulty of using the English language. That is, public and patient education are seen by many doctors as an extension of public health, a discipline that is tangential to the daily concerns of practicing physicians. Public health is designed to keep healthy people from becoming sick. The reward for success in this domain, therefore, is that *nothing happens*—people don't get sick; to most physicians, preventing sickness, however laudable in theory, lacks the intellectual challenge (not to mention the social and financial rewards) of making sick people better—which is, after all, what doctors are trained to do. So it is, for example, that physicians generate more enthusiasm for tracking down causes and treating infection in acutely ill patients than they do about getting people to wash their hands or to use condoms, to prevent infection in the first place. It's worth noting in this regard that nurses' perspective tilts toward caring more than toward curing, while for physicians it's generally the other way around. It can hardly be an accident, then, that nurses take patient and public education so seriously, spend so much time at it, and often may even be better at it than physicians.

And there is a darker side: the issue of control. For all its healing and cooperative aspects, the relationship between doctors and patients inevitably also involves establishing and maintaining a degree of control on both sides. For a long time, the balance of control lay mainly with physicians, largely because they controlled the giving of information and because they withheld it, as, for example, when they spoke or wrote their prescriptions in Latin. The balance of control has shifted progressively toward the patient side in recent years, but as recently as the 1970s, the great majority of practicing physicians still explicitly supported the ancient medical tradition of withholding information (e.g., a diagnosis of cancer) from patients (3).

These reflections explain some of the difficulties the medical profession has had with patient and public education; they also suggest that changing the situation will be an uphill struggle. Some thoughts follow on steps that might help.

First, it is useful to distinguish between *public* and *patient* education: The educational needs and expectations of the two groups are different, and require different approaches and techniques. Public education focuses on people in groups who aren't sick or don't think of themselves as patients, and, where the need exists for wide dissemination of information, it focuses primarily on prevention. *Patient* education, in contrast, is aimed at specific, individual people who have entered the patient role because of symptoms or diagnosed diseases. Here the need is for information delivered within a professional relationship and tailored to individual circumstance.

A second step is to recognize that prevention goes well beyond the narrow public health definition associated with things like maintaining clean water supplies or using seat belts. The concept of prevention was usefully broadened some years ago to include *primary* (removing risk-producing exposures from still-healthy people), *secondary* (early detection and treatment of presymptomatic disease), and *tertiary* (interventions in symptomatic patients that reduce recurrence and prevent disability) varieties (4). Prevention thus legitimately spans both public and patient education and enters nearly every phase of clinical medicine. From this broader perspective, clinical tasks like management of osteopenia in individual patients consist principally of secondary prevention (5), and education of women at menopause about estrogen replacement is just as much prevention as education about hand-washing or vaccination.

A third step is to expect physicians to teach only what is worth teaching. Public education isn't free; it requires time, money, expertise. Moreover, public education creates public expectations which, in certain areas like mass screening, can consume huge amounts of medical resources. Good public education, therefore, like good medicine in general, should be evidence based (6). And although the evidence for a number of preventive practices is still controversial (e.g., mammographic screening of women below age 50 for breast cancer), clear-cut evidence regarding the effectiveness, or lack of it, of many preventive practices is now available (7).

A fourth step is to be aware that, even when the rationale and evidence for preventive practices are clear and compelling, patient education and preventive care can get lost in the shuffle unless the system of care is specifically organized to support these activities. An office that has flow sheets in patient records, automated reminders (8), and smoothly functioning referral systems, for example, is more likely to implement patient education and effective preventive practices than one that doesn't.

A fifth step is to accept the importance of learning *how* to teach patients well. Just because someone is good at taking medical histories, listening to hearts, and the like does not mean they will necessarily be good at teaching patients or motivating them to take better care of themselves. Powerful models for effective counseling now exist. The logic of good medical practice requires that physicians learn those models and the specific skills associated with them at least as well as they learn the pathophysiological models and the management techniques for specific diseases.

Physicians underestimate the enormous therapeutic power they can exercise through patient and public education, a power that the British psychiatrist Michael Balint likened to that of a pharmaceutical agent, referring to it as "the drug 'doctor'" (9). For example, smokers will quit in significant numbers if their physicians simply advise them to, but not all physicians do so. (See Chapter 20, Quitting.) Physicians use the drug doctor at full strength when they educate their patients and the public effectively.

REFERENCES

1. **Cohn V.** News and Numbers. Ames, IA: Iowa State University Press; 1989.
2. **Smith T.** Information for patients. Writing simple English is difficult, even for doctors. BMJ. 1992;305:1242.
3. **Laine C, Davidoff F.** Patient-centered medicine: a professional evolution. JAMA. 1996;275:152-6.
4. **Mausner JS, Bahn AK.** Epidemiology: An Introductory Text. Philadelphia: WB Saunders; 1974.
5. **Riggs BL, Melton LJ III.** The prevention and treatment of osteoporosis. N Engl J Med. 1992;327:620-7.
6. **Evidence-Based Medicine Working Group.** Evidence-based medicine. A new approach to teaching the practice of medicine. JAMA. 1992;268:2420-5.
7. **U.S. Preventive Services Task Force.** Guide to Clinical Preventive Services. An assessment of the effectiveness of 169 interventions: Report of the U.S. Preventive Services Task Force. Baltimore: Williams and Wilkins; 1989.
8. **McDonald CJ, Sui SL, Smith DM, Tierney WM, Cohen SJ, Weinberger M, et al.** Reminders to physicians from an introspective computer medical record. A two-year randomized trial. Ann Intern Med. 1984;100:130-4.
9. **Balint M.** The Doctor, His Patient, and the Illness. New York: International Universities Press; 1972.

CHAPTER 39

The Best of All Worlds

Medical Education in the Global Village

The year was 1946. Europe was just starting to rebuild itself from the ashes of World War II. My father, a neurosurgeon, was invited to join a WHO/American Friends Service Committee medical teaching mission to Czechoslovakia, helping physicians in that war-ravaged country back into the mainstream of western medicine after their long isolation. The trip demanded many hours of teaching on rounds and in the operating room, but produced, among other memorable results, a pilgrimage to Gregor Mendel's house, a medal (the Order of the White Lion) from the Czech government, much camaraderie, and several long-standing trans-Atlantic friendships. The mission undoubtedly helped Czech medicine at least a little, but the style and scale of this effort are certainly more reminiscent of "The Grand Illusion" than "Apocalypse Now."

Cut to 1992. I am given an elegant brochure for the International Medical College, a new medical school in Kuala Lumpur, Malaysia. Created jointly by some of the world's leading medical educators from Malaysia, the United States, Canada, Ireland, Scotland, England, Australia, and New Zealand, the school will train students for the entire Southeast Asian region, and will be run as a partnership among faculty from these countries. Students will spend their three introductory, mostly preclinical, years in Malaysia learning in a highly sophisticated educational environment that includes task-based learning, a flexible core curriculum, assessment-to-a-standard rather than fixed-length

211

courses, a notebook personal computer for every student, and a rigorous examination system that evaluates clinical skills as well as knowledge. The student's clinical years will be spent in a partner medical school overseas. Welcome to the medical education global village.

Unfortunately, despite the rapid and progressive globalization of everything from diseases and economies to cooking and music, the kind of dazzling, state-of-the-art international medical education promised by the nascent Malaysian school remains the exception rather than the rule. Why have the globalization of medicine and medical education lagged so far behind? For one thing, medical need is closely tied to economic development which, of course, varies enormously from country to country. Thus, in the developing world, the dominant need is in preventive and population medicine, particularly related to infectious and nutritional disease, which, in turn, are closely tied to problems of sanitation, food supply, and housing. The problem is that medicine in these countries is tempted to leapfrog over the clinical essentials and on into high-technology medicine, even when high-tech medicine isn't the best match between resources and needs and when the technology can't be adequately supported or maintained. In the so-called "transition" countries, with somewhat stronger and more industrialized economies, the worst of the poverty-driven health problems have been dealt with, but the diseases of the developed world—chronic illness, diseases of the elderly—are rapidly becoming more prevalent (1). And, of course, in developed countries, medical needs are not so very different from those found in the United States.

For another thing, medicine, whether operating at a relatively undeveloped level or at its scientific best, is principally a social act. This means that in every country, the social meaning of illness, of medical practice, and of medical teaching itself are all closely tied to, and vary with, local social and cultural realities. While the universals of human biology do make it possible to share some aspects of medicine and medical teaching across international boundaries, many aspects of medical practice or teaching will be hard to export, since their introduction would require major changes in the social process, which may be neither easy nor desirable.

As an example, medical educators from the west were consulted recently by a group of medical schools in mainland China for help in improving undergraduate clinical teaching. The consultants noticed, among other things, that the tubing on the medical students' stethoscopes was very long, which made auscultation difficult and frustrating (longer tubing transmits sound less well than shorter tubing). On investigation, it turned out that the length of the tubing was not accidental, but was intended to preserve the socially acceptable distance between patient and caregiver. While it took time, the consultants eventually managed to get stethoscope tubing shortened, through a combination of diplomacy and explanations about the physics of sound (2). As another example, the importance of continuing professional education and development is not taken for granted in many countries, including China, to the extent it is in others. And although that perception is beginning to change, the challenges of creating an expanded and effective CME system in many countries are daunting.

A full and free trade of the best the world has to offer in medical education is an attractive vision, but in this particular commerce, as in so many others, a balance of trade (so to speak) between the United States and the rest of the world is important, despite the many potential barriers to achieving it. On the export side, there are the many basic but crucial education and information resources whose availability we take for granted here but that are in terribly short supply abroad. Perhaps the most pressing need of this kind is for medical publications, since physicians are often paid so little they can't afford their own subscriptions, and hospital and medical school libraries in many countries are hurting badly for hard currency. And while English is nearly a universal medical language, it is principally the academic physicians in many countries who are fluent, while practitioners are less well equipped in this regard. An obvious solution to this latter problem is to translate, publish, and distribute journals in languages other than English (or other original languages). Unfortunately, the logistic and economic obstacles to producing translated editions are formidable. What's more, the medical leadership in non–English-speaking countries doesn't uniformly support translation of medical texts into their own language, since the use of languages other than English in medical communication is seen as retrogressive, something that separates local physicians from the larger world medical community.

Expertise in the design and organization of CME programs can also be a valuable U.S. educational export. Many potential consumer countries still have modest or even rudimentary CME programs. The prospect of helping people in those countries produce programs that meet local needs is therefore attractive, particularly if, at the same time, it helps them avoid the worst mistakes we have made as we created our own CME enterprise. For want of better information, for example, educators in many countries have sometimes assumed that CME credit exists in one form only—the time-based and hour-for-hour found in the United States and elsewhere. But time-based, hour-for-hour credit can be constraining, even counterproductive, and effective, more rational alternatives to time-based credit exist (see Chapter 37, Units of Learning, Not Units of Teaching); it would be appropriate, and perhaps more ethical, to support the development of alternative forms of credit in countries seeking to develop their CME credit systems anew.

Education about the appropriate use of at least some new technologies may be an important export—from the use of notebook computers by medical students in Kuala Lumpur, to the use of ultrasound at the university hospital in Lahore. Whether medical educators should support the export of the technologies themselves is another question altogether.

Finally, the United States and other developed countries have for years exported medical expertise. Some of this happens when individual faculty from a donor country participate in knowledge update courses or congresses outside their own borders. This sort of involvement can result in professional, social, and political benefits that are substantial, although the educational effectiveness of such programs is highly questionable. (See Chapter 30, Does Continuing Medical Education Work?, and Chapter 35, Managing Messes.) Expertise is also exported when physicians from the United States and elsewhere serve as visiting faculty in residence in other countries, usually for short periods (i.e., days to weeks, or, less often, for months or even years). Experience suggests that short-term service generally benefits the visiting physician more than the host institution, but the balance shifts progressively toward the institution as the length of the stay increases.

The export of expertise from the developed world takes place principally, however, when young physicians trained initially in their home countries in the developing world undertake further residency or fellowship training in the United States or elsewhere, then return to their country of origin. While this export has undoubtedly contributed to the improvement of medicine in the developing world, many of these highly trained people encounter daunting social and economic barriers when they try to put their special training to work after they return (3). Finding ways to support their careers in their home institutions remains an important challenge, but there are already a few highly successful examples in existence, such as the Rockefeller Foundation–supported International Clinical Epidemiology Network (INCLEN), that can serve as models.

A healthy medical education balance of trade of course requires imports as well as exports, and, in this connection, it is fortunate for all concerned that both the quantity and quality of such imports into the United States are on the rise. First, of course, the United States already imports a great deal of physician manpower into our residencies, which then moves on out into our practice community. These physicians bring with them an enormous richness and diversity, both cultural and medical. For example, physicians who obtain their initial training in a variety of other countries, including South Africa and New Zealand, usually develop bedside clinical skills that far outstrip those of most U.S. physicians; we have a lot to learn from them. Second, as we increasingly confront the reality that the U.S. health care system, for all its strengths, is seriously flawed, we discover that people in other countries have a great deal to teach us about efficient and effective medical care delivery (4).

Third, the results of clinical research imported from other countries increasingly inform our medical teaching: For example, an increasing number of well-designed clinical trials on key medical questions are made possible only through international cooperation among many participating researchers and institutions (5). And witness the substantial and growing proportion of manuscripts from abroad submitted to and published by major U.S. medical journals: over 25 percent of the 2,400 manuscripts submitted each year to the *Annals of Internal Medicine,* many of extremely high quality, now come from countries outside the United States. Researchers and teachers from non–U.S. medical schools increasingly participate as faculty in some of our best CME programs. And there is little doubt that the explosive development of the Internet has helped medical educators and researchers from all over the world to work together: faster, more efficiently, and on a more equal footing. Finally, a number of important innovations that have affected medical thinking, research and education in the United States—from the Objective Structured Clinical Examination (OSCE), to problem-based learning and community-oriented medical school curriculum, to the international Cochrane Collaboration—either originated in, or received major developmental impetus from, the medical teachers and researchers of other countries (6–8).

On reflection, it's clear we've come a very long way in international medical education from post–World War II medical missions. The sharing of the best the world has to offer in medical education may, in fact, be a lot greater than we've been willing to admit. But for all we've learned and shared in medical education, we haven't quite become a medical global village, at least not yet.

REFERENCES

1. **Escovitz G.** The health transition in developing countries. Ann Intern Med. 1992;116:499-504.
2. **Stillman PL, Sawyer WD.** A new program to enhance the teaching and assessment of clinical skills in the People's Republic of China. Acad Med. 1992;67:495-9.
3. **Patel V, Araya R.** Trained overseas, unable to return home: plight of doctors from developing countries. Lancet. 1992;339:110-1.
4. **Iglehart JK.** Germany's health care system. N Engl J Med. 1991;324:503-8 [Part 1]; 1750-6 [Part 2].
5. **Neilson JP.** Magnesium sulphate: the drug of choice in eclampsia. BMJ. 1995;311:702-3.
6. **White KL, Connelly JE, eds.** The Medical School's Mission and the Population's Health: Medical Education in Canada, the United Kingdom, the United States, and Australia. New York: Springer-Verlag; 1992.
7. **Schmidt HG, Lipkin M Jr, deVries MW, Greep JM, eds.** New Directions for Medical Education. Problem-Based Learning and Community-Oriented Medical Education. New York: Springer-Verlag; 1989.
8. **Chalmers I.** The Cochrane Collaboration: preparing, maintaining, and disseminating systematic reviews of the effects of health care. Ann N Y Acad Sci. 1993;703:156-63.

CHAPTER 40

Push and Pull

~

Joining Recertification and Continuing Medical Education

With recertification in internal medicine now a reality (1), it has become increasingly important to understand just where CME leaves off and recertification begins, and the relationship—both the synergy and the tension—between the two.

The idea of recertification isn't new. Specialty board certification, which began in 1917, was one of the earliest formal medical standard setting–mechanisms in this country, and has come to enjoy wide respect. While at the beginning, certificates in all specialties were awarded without limit of time, the American Board of Medical Specialties (the umbrella organization of the specialty boards) as early as 1936 had already raised questions about the validity of "once and for all" certification, and suggested the possibility of recertification "at stipulated intervals." It was not, however, until the American Board of Family Practice did so in 1969 that a medical specialty actually set a time limit on certification (2), thus making recertification a reality. Since then, virtually all of the medical specialty boards have begun to issue time-limited certificates, or have plans to do so.

Time-limited certification is not, of course, synonymous with recertification, but a time limit on board certificates obviously creates the need for recertification, since physicians would otherwise remain uncertified in their specialty after the time limit on their certificates ran out. In the 1970s, the American Board of Internal Medicine (ABIM) offered several recertification programs on a voluntary basis, that is, without making initial certification time limited. ABIM later abandoned the voluntary approach because less than 5 percent of eligible internists were pulled into the process, a disappointing but perhaps not surprising outcome in view of the lack of push from time limitation.

Recertification is now uniformly linked to time-limited initial certification across specialties. Moreover, all boards seem to have independently adopted certain elements in common as they designed their recertification programs: an expectation, formal or informal, of continued scholarship; maintenance of medical licensure; some form of clinical practice or performance evaluation, usually local; and a written examination, which is mostly proctored, timed, and secured, although in some instances an open book or take-home (self-assessment) examination is also included.

At the same time, the various boards have taken a variety of approaches to certain other aspects of recertification. Particularly intriguing is the variation among specialties in the way the elements of recertification and education have been shared out between the board in each specialty and its respective professional society. In pediatrics, for example, the board and the academy initially forged a formal Joint Committee whose purpose was "to develop a program of education and evaluation which would be guided by common objectives" (3). Their procedure was to write pools of multiple-choice questions based on specific educational objectives, then parcel out these questions either to the evaluation or the education side of the program. Despite the later dissolution of the Joint Committee and the formal relationship, the two arms of the enterprise have continued working fairly closely together. The board and the college of obstetrics and gynecology collaborate in similar fashion, but in other specialties, the working relationships between boards and professional societies have been more limited as recertification programs have been developed.

Specialty certification is primarily "summative," so called because it summarizes the status of a candidate's knowledge, and, to some degree, competence, at the end of a period of training and experience. Specialty education, in contrast, is primarily "formative," because it forms trainees' knowledge and competencies, preparing them for practice in that specialty (as well as preparing them for the certification examinations that serve as one surrogate measure of practice competence).

Thus, while initial certification and education ultimately converge on the same goal of professional excellence, the two come at the task by means of very different approaches. These differences are obvious enough to create an expectation that relatively simple, clear lines will separate those who certify and recertify from those who educate, but the mix of shared goals plus independent means to those goals has in actuality led to complex and subtle "arms length" yet codependent relationships between the two groups. Thus, for example, the principal CME organization of internists, the American College of Physicians, was one of the founders of the ABIM, and worked closely with the board in the 1930s and '40s to develop the initial certification process. For at least thirty years, therefore, specialty certificates in internal medicine carried the names of both organizations; the two also collaborated in developing the voluntary recertification programs of the 1970s. Moreover, the ACP's Medical Knowledge Self-Assessment Program, which has been nominally developed to evaluate and update the knowledge of practicing internists, is widely used by residents in preparing for the board examination.

Conversely, while the ABIM has consistently and consciously distanced itself from the education of medical residents, it has exerted, and continues to exert, enormous influence on that education. It does so through its hospital and program visits, its definitions of clinical competence and the like, and its support of hospital accreditation (residents are not board-eligible unless the hospital in which they are trained is accredited). Most importantly, the ABIM, as one of the three sitting "parents" of the Residency Review Committee in Internal Medicine, helps to shape the standards and practices of the very residency programs that lead to board eligibility, including (among other things) the elements of curriculum, the nature of teaching rounds, expected board participation and pass rates, and the length of residency training.

Despite the years of interaction between the ABIM and the residency education system around issues of *initial certification*, it is difficult to predict how *recertification* will affect CME and vice versa, since the circumstances surrounding initial certification and recertification aren't exactly parallel. Still, given the march of events leading to recertification, some educated guesses may be permitted even now. CME in the United States arguably still operates in a "pre-Flexnerian" mode; it is fragmented and geographically dispersed, inefficient and inconsistent in quality, and fairly heavily commercialized, thus closely resembling the American medical schools of the nineteenth and early twentieth centuries. This state of affairs has not been lost on the creators of recertification, who believe that "without a test, CME really has no clout. It doesn't function effectively" (4). As a result, they have taken the position that "if the recertification process does nothing more than stimulate a renewed study pattern it is accomplishing its goal" (5). Recertification's principal effect on CME might, therefore, be simply quantitative: that is, it may stimulate more of the same CME. But while an increase in amount might be useful, the more important effect would be qualitative: Recertification might make CME better, for example, by catalyzing improvements in CME methods and standards, by giving CME increased focus and salience.

In the last analysis, there is little doubt that recertification will affect CME; it is largely a question of when, how, and how much. The effects, paradoxically, could play out in at least two opposing ways. In one scenario, recertification's clout could become so great that formal CME credit would become irrelevant, and the entire CME enterprise as we know it would fade into the sunset. In a contrary scenario, recertification could render CME and CME credit more meaningful than ever because it would create a powerful summative mechanism, the kind of force that formal national evaluation systems always provide for education, but one which does not now exist for practicing physicians.

In the optimal scenario, the interactions between CME and recertification would be close, active, and mutually reinforcing. In other words, a strong recertification process can and should influence CME for the better and, equally important, stronger CME should strengthen recertification; stimulating CME is, after all, one of the explicit goals of recertification. Indeed, the advent of recertification presents the ABIM, the CME organizations, and internists in general with an enormous, perhaps a one-time, opportunity. Given ABIM's active and positive track record in resident education—the process that leads to initial Board certification—a similarly active involvement of ABIM in the CME process seems not only logical but necessary, both in CME standard setting and in the application of those standards. At the same time, the internal medicine CME organizations will need to reciprocate if both recertification and CME are to realize their full potential. In the recertification era, the individual hands of recertification and of CME can exert considerable positive force on professional competence and, ultimately, patient care, even if the two pull separately. Their effectiveness could be greatly magnified, however, if the two hands pull together.

REFERENCES

1. **Glassock RJ, Benson JA Jr, Copeland RB, Godwin HA Jr, Johanson WG Jr, Point W, et al.** Time-limited certification and recertification:

the program of the American Board of Internal Medicine. The Task Force on Recertification. Ann Intern Med. 1992;114:59-62.
2. **Lloyd JS.** History and present status of recertification. In: Lloyd JS, Langsley DG, eds. Recertification for Medical Specialists. Evanston, IL: American Board of Medical Specialties; 1987:3-10.
3. **Brownlee RC.** Recertification examinations linked to CME. In: Lloyd JS, Langsley DG, eds. Recertification for Medical Specialists. Evanston, IL: American Board of Medical Specialties; 1987:43-8.
4. **Jaffe BM.** Pros and cons of time-limited certification. In: Lloyd JS, Langsley DG, eds. Recertification for Medical Specialists. Evanston, IL: American Board of Medical Specialties; 1987:59-62.
5. **Griffin JO Jr.** Time-limited certification. In: Lloyd JS, Langsley DG, eds. Recertification for Medical Specialists. Evanston, IL: American Board of Medical Specialties; 1987:37-42.

CHAPTER *41*

Changing Times, Changing Careers

Transformation and Education

[with Kathleen L. Egan, PhD]

*T*he medical world in the United States is changing: from fee-for-service to capitation; from private practice to managed care; from unaccountable to profiled; from a push toward subspecialization to a move toward generalism. The upheaval seems to have taken on a momentum of its own, pulling and tumbling us along with it. And at the epicenter of the changes are physicians, many of whom are experiencing or expecting fundamental alterations in their lives and work. A health care system that is "wringing out" an oversupply of highly specialized physicians (1) is already pushing some specialists and subspecialists, inside internal medicine and outside it, to make the shift to a new and more general career direction, thereby creating the need to undertake the kind of education that supports this career change.

While much of the widespread talk about these issues makes *retraining* (and its more palatable label *career change*) seem like a new phenomenon, the reality is that physicians have always made changes in career direction, albeit in relatively small numbers. Some have added areas of special competence, for instance; others have moved into or out of research. A few have made more drastic changes, for example, to an entirely new specialty or even out of medicine altogether and into business, politics, or administration. Re-education for a new kind of medical career is therefore not exactly a new idea.

In extensive interviews with 340 physicians in the United States and Canada, Fox and his colleagues found that for physicians who decide to undergo this most profound kind of change—what Fox has called transformation (2)—the trigger for change was frequently a negative event such as ill health or rapidly increasing stress (2). As the authors report, "The typical statement was not 'it seemed like a fine opportunity so I . . .' but rather, 'the situation was so difficult that I . . .' " (2, p 46). Yet in the end, the outcomes for many of these changes were positive. One physician described his decision to cut out a major part of his practice and spend more time at home after suffering a myocardial infarction this way: "You know, I didn't expect anything positive to come from a heart attack at my age . . . but it did (2, p 45)." From another source comes a description of an internist who found his real earnings flat over a three-year period and "threw in the towel." He became a salaried employee of a health care corporation, and he reports that his compensation will rise almost 50 percent while he is no longer responsible for the headaches of running an office (3).

But large, complex changes such as these involve major restructuring of one's entire professional life, along with significant new learning, and are associated with strong, not always pleasant, emotions. And the work of Fox and colleagues discovered that while both external pressures and physicians' emotional state were most often responsible for inciting the change, the actual process of changing involved organized, information-based thought that interacted with these emotions and attitudes. Learning new information and skills contributed to the change in some two thirds of the study sample (2, p 47), and learning helped determine the quality and character of the change (2, p 48). For those who make the change, the challenge, therefore, is how to undertake the kind of drastic re-education that will best support the transformation. That education needs to be as close to the ideal as possible; change is difficult enough as it is, without the associated education being ineffective or, even worse, burdensome.

Educators have long recognized that what distinguishes education from simple information transfer is that education, by definition, results in change, while information may or may not. (See Chapter 2, Information and Education.) But education-related change requires motivation, and Deci and colleagues (4) have argued convincingly that education motivates learners to change when it supports *autonomy*, creates *connectedness*, and leads to *mastery*. The sort of learning experiences that minimize the disruptions of career change and make transformative moves as productive as possible—in a word, education approaching the ideal for this unusual group—will therefore need to pay careful attention to the group's particular needs for autonomy, connectedness, and mastery.

AUTONOMY

In support of autonomy, education related to career change should be *collaborative,* a joint endeavor among learners, peers, and faculty, respecting the weight and value of the participating physicians' clinical experience and the collegial character of medicine. For example, the physician-learners should be active partners in identifying what needs to be taught and learned. They should be given the opportunity to assess what they are already comfortable with and what additional skills and information are needed for success in the new practice context.

In similar fashion, including physician-learners in the periodic evaluation of their own learning is likely to produce more meaningful insights than judgments by a teacher or mentor alone. These learners are, after all, likely to be "reflective practitioners" already, in Schön's terms (5), adept at mentally reviewing their own performance and identifying how it might be improved next time. When combined with the insights of additional faculty and peers, autonomy-supporting assessments such as these are likely to pay off by substantially accelerating and smoothing the transition to a new professional identity and by increasing physicians' effectiveness in their new role.

CONNECTEDNESS

To establish connectedness, programs in career change education will need to provide opportunities for physicians to join colleagues who are undergoing the same or similar transformative experiences. Linkages like this can be critical for learning, support, and verification of experience, and for offsetting the feeling of isolation from the previous subspecialty or practice colleagues. Physicians undertaking major shifts in career direction are also likely to experience a loss of collegiality with and status among their peers. Mentors are therefore crucial in guiding physician-learners' exploration of new roles, and helping to identify peers with whom to compare experiences and colleagues for mutual support. A wide variety of studies inform us that interactions with colleagues and consultants are among the most frequently used, attractive, and effective forms of learning for practicing clinicians. The "College Within a College," a small-group, collegial approach to learning at the

American College of Physicians' own Annual Session bears this out. Participants use the large meeting as a resource to teach and learn directly from each other. Over several years, they have found it effective, and vastly more congenial that attendance on one's own.

MASTERY

At a recent national meeting on continuing medical education, a representative of the Pew Commission on Health Professions challenged the continuing medical education community to focus "retraining" for generalist careers on the mastery of *new* competencies. Learning for this particular career change is not at all a matter of "getting back to basics" or a downgrading of skills. On the contrary, this learning should be substantive, allowing new and higher mastery to emerge: dealing with the uncertainties of undifferentiated problems; managing multiproblem patients; dealing with whatever the patient brings and doing so in a way that is sensitive to the context of the patient's life. Looked at this way, generalism is at least as advanced, complex, and sophisticated as any of the medical subspecialty disciplines.

Generalists will also be called on increasingly to take on new roles on health care teams, as coach and mentor, and in organizations, for example, as leader in quality improvement, in evaluating and adapting practice guidelines and clinical pathways, and in shaping health care organizations so that they keep the quality of care and patients outcomes in the forefront. Ideally, then, generalist career change education should lead to the creation of a cohort of particularly sophisticated and creative physicians positioned to lead and shape the rapidly evolving health care system. Since the transforming specialist or subspecialist may be feeling the loss of hard-won mastery of high-level knowledge and skill, the sense that there are new concepts and abilities worth attaining, and that there is real and important new work for them to do, will be highly valued.

In sum, for career change education to be useful in transformative career change, it will need to be designed in ways that meet the special requirements of these special learners. It cannot be simply an adaptation of medical or residency experiences but must be a thing unto itself. And it must take full advantage of the best of what we know about supporting and motivating people during these often wrenching transitions.

Change always involves both losses and gains; the Chinese ideogram for change contains symbols for both danger and opportunity. Thus, early in the realization that a coming change is inevitable, people understandably tend to be oriented to the past and present: defending and protecting the past, trying to maintain the present, and denying the emerging reality—somewhat like patients dealing with the reality of fatal illness (6).

For many physicians, the career changes they are facing already or will soon face may, in fact, feel like the death of professional life and practice as they have known it. Once it becomes possible to move to, and then beyond, the stages of resignation and acceptance, however, transformative change of the most positive kind becomes a possibility. We owe it to both ourselves and our patients to handle the coming shakeout in medical careers in ways that deal effectively with losses and transform them into gains.

REFERENCES

1. **Weiner J.** Forecasting the effects of health care reform on U.S. physician work force requirement. Evidence from HMO staffing patterns. JAMA. 1994;272:222-30.
2. **Fox RD, Mazmanian PE, Putnam RW.** Changing and Learning in the Lives of Physicians. New York: Praeger; 1989.
3. **Walsh M.** Doctors signing on as employees, not looking back. Forbes Magazine, July 4, 1994, p. 58 as cited in Report on Physician Trends, Vol. 2, No. 8, August 1994.
4. **Deci EI, Valelrand RJ, Pelletier LG, Ryan RM.** Motivation and education: the self-determination perspective. Educational Psychologist. 1991;26:325-46.
5. **Schön D.** Educating the Reflective Practitioner. Toward a New Design for Teaching and Learning in the Professions. San Francisco: Jossey-Bass; 1987.
6. **Kubler-Ross E.** On Death and Dying. New York: The Macmillan Co.; 1969.

INDEX